MW00778472

GROWING MARIJUANA INDOORS

A Foolproof Guide

GROWING MARIJUANA *Indoors*

A FOOLPROOF GUIDE

by JAY CARTER BROWN

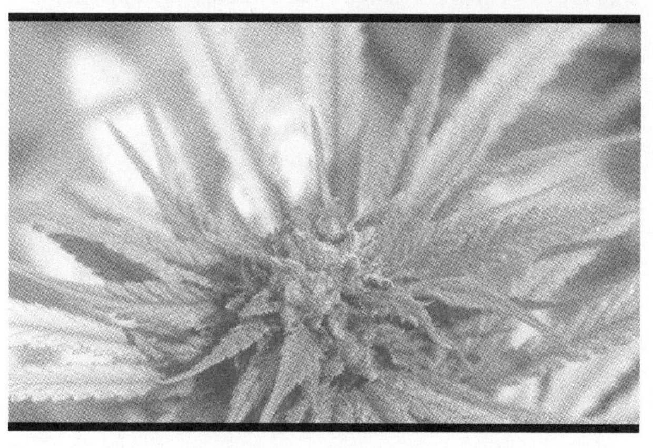

ECW PRESS

Published by ECW Press
2120 Queen Street East, Suite 200, Toronto, Ontario, Canada M4E 1E2
416-694-3348 / info@ecwpress.com

LIBRARY AND ARCHIVES CANADA CATALOGUING IN PUBLICATION

Brown, Jay Carter
Growing marijuana indoors : a foolproof guide / Jay Carter Brown.

ISBN 978-1-77041-129-6
Also issued as: 978-1-77090-375-3 (PDF); 978-1-77090-376-0 (EPUB)

1. Marijuana. 2. Cannabis. I. Title.

SB295.C35B76 2013 633.7'9 C2012-907525-6

Cover and text design: Natalie Olsen, Kisscut Design
All images courtesy of the author
Printing: United Graphics 5 4 3 2 1

Printed and bound in the United States

I dedicate this book to my wife
who has stayed with me through
thick and thin, for richer or poorer,
in sickness and in health

CONTENTS

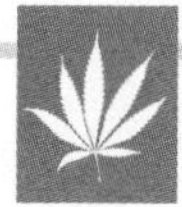

Introduction

I wrote this book for my wife. We both smoke cannabis and have done so for most of our lives. When I started buying cannabis, it was almost affordable if you smoked less than an ounce a month. But once you went beyond that amount, it was prudent to find some other way of obtaining "the weed." Some people dealt a little weed and subsidized their habit that way. Others smuggled large amounts of herb into the country and pulled a bale out for their own use. Today both solutions can lead to hard time and financial ruin under North America's seizure and forfeiture statutes.

In Canada, people can legally obtain a license to use medical marijuana if they follow the correct steps. On the surface, this appears to be an intelligent way of obtaining marijuana. But there is no guarantee that a person will be approved for medical marijuana since most doctors refuse to sign off on the appropriate government forms, perhaps from fear of reprisals.

Even if people are approved to possess marijuana, they might still have to pay someone to grow it for them. (Pot in Vancouver compassion clubs is currently about $10 per gram, which is around the same price or higher than it costs on the street.) A cannabis growing license is even harder to get than a cannabis possession license. Growing pot can be done legally in Canada with a government permit that allows a patient or a designated third party to grow cannabis. Those who wish to apply for a permit in Canada can visit the Health Canada website for medical marijuana access or write to Marihuana Medical Access Division, Drug Strategy and Controlled Substance Programme, Health Canada, Address Locator 3503B, Ottawa, Ontario, K1A 1B9.

In a dozen or more states in America, there are similar programs at the state level. Federal law in the United States opposes a state's right to dispense marijuana or issue marijuana growing permits, but more states are defying the Feds on this front. In fact in 2012 both Washington and Colorado voted to decriminalize the use of non-medical (recreational) marijuana. My own feelings are mixed about the growing permit solution because I have never trusted governments. They often change or reverse their thinking, and if that happens where does it leave pot growers who have applied for a medical pot license? It's too late to grow your pot surreptitiously once you have already outed yourself to the government. For that reason, in the past I have used most of the generally known methods to access pot, including smuggling, dealing, and growing (outdoor and indoor, in soil, as well as with hydroponics).

Growing Marijuana Indoors outlines my preferred method of growing marijuana, one I have synthesized from my decades of experience growing pot. If you follow my rules exactly, my system is fail proof — so fail proof that it could be called "Pot Growing for Dummies." But since this book is primarily for my wife, I won't call it that! The idea behind this handbook was that, if for whatever reason I am not around, my wife can decide for herself if she wants her "medicine" without having to rely on anyone else to get it for her. Follow the steps laid out in this book to the letter, and you'll have success at growing the finest marijuana that even money can't buy.

Peace and love to everyone.

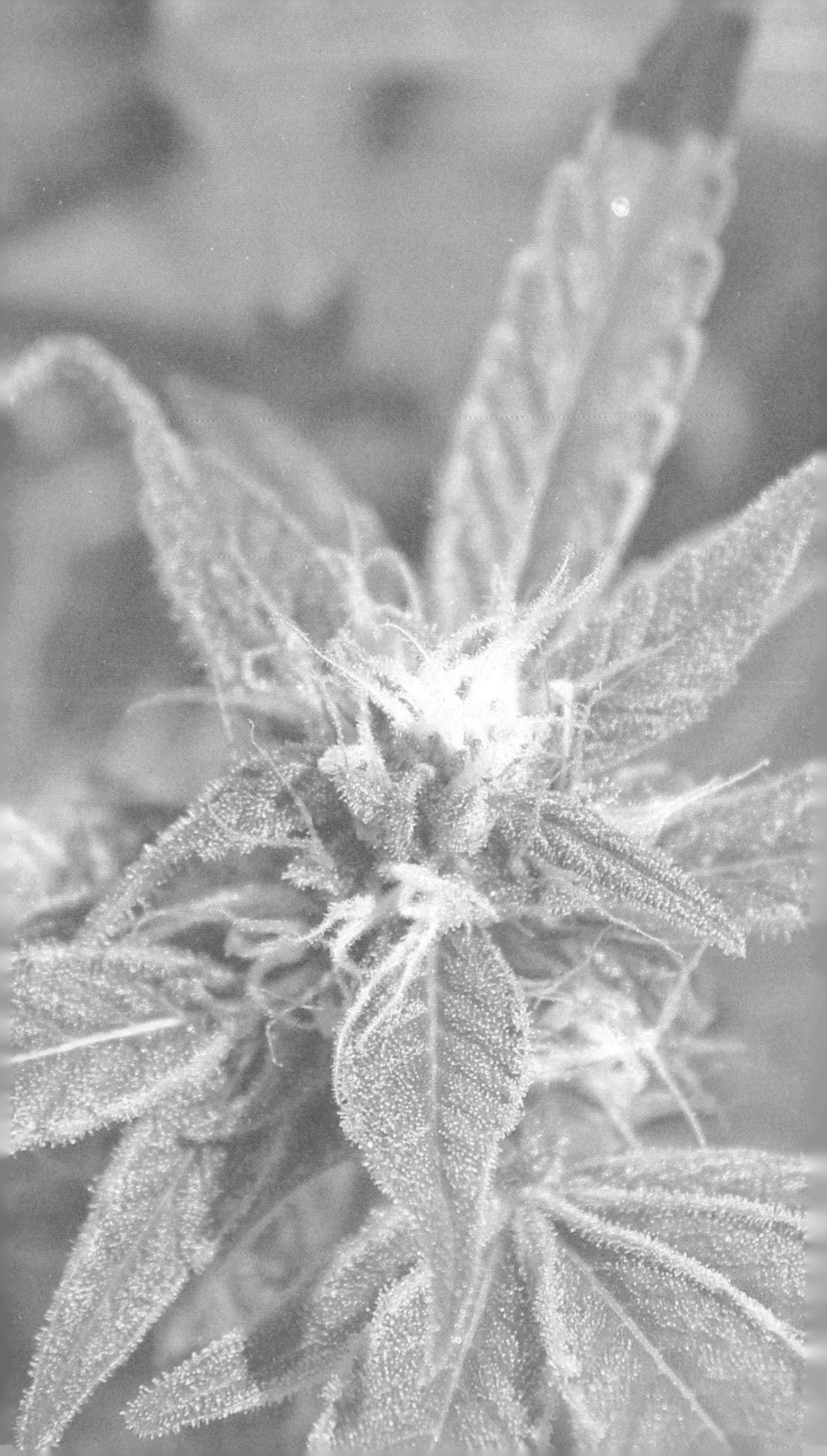

1

PREPARING *for* YOUR GARDEN

Marijuana 101

Conventional wisdom says that it is easy to grow marijuana. It is said to be a weed and, as such, grows anywhere and everywhere without any help from humans. This might have been true at one time but only to a point. Marijuana has been cultivated throughout history and was carried by humans wherever they went, so it didn't grow wild on its own accord for long. Weed was always too valuable to be left wild and free without someone harvesting it and taking advantage of its bounty. Therefore, most cannabis in the world today is the result of careful breeding and gardening techniques. Wild marijuana is said to taste better than cultivated marijuana, but when grown indoors the wild variety is skinny and weak compared with designer-bred indoor strains. Although any type of pot can be grown indoors, every effort must be made to find the best genetic strain that will compensate for the disadvantages of indoor cultivation and be adaptable to lighting that is far weaker than the sun.

Indoor weed is bred to provide the best results for cannabis grown under lights, and it usually begins with an Indica strain. Cannabis Indica is the variety of marijuana used to make hashish. Indica plants grow shorter and thicker and provide stronger highs than the alternate variety of marijuana known as Cannabis Sativa. In effect, indoor Sativa is not a true Sativa plant at all. It is an Indica plant crossbred with a Sativa plant for an airier high. Pure Sativa plants do very poorly indoors. They take longer to grow and are skinnier and less potent than Indica plants. But Sativa plants can provide a soaring mental high without the drag-down effects of the sleep-inducing Indica plants. Therefore, crossbreeding can provide the best features of both plants, and it can be very rewarding to breed your own special brand of marijuana based on your preference for taste, potency, quality of high, long-lasting effects, burning qualities, and so on.

Male cannabis plants produce flowers that pollinate the female cannabis buds but offer very little THC, which is the active ingredient in cannabis that makes you high. Only the female plant is used to produce the dried flowers known as cannabis, but it is not the branches or leaves or buds that make you high, it is the tiny capitate-stalked trichomes or THC crystals that grow on the branches, leaves, and buds. So you are not really harvesting buds, you are harvesting the trichomes/crystals that cover the buds. It is possible to harvest some THC crystals from the leaves and branches of both the female and male cannabis plants, but not in sufficient quantities to make for good smoking.

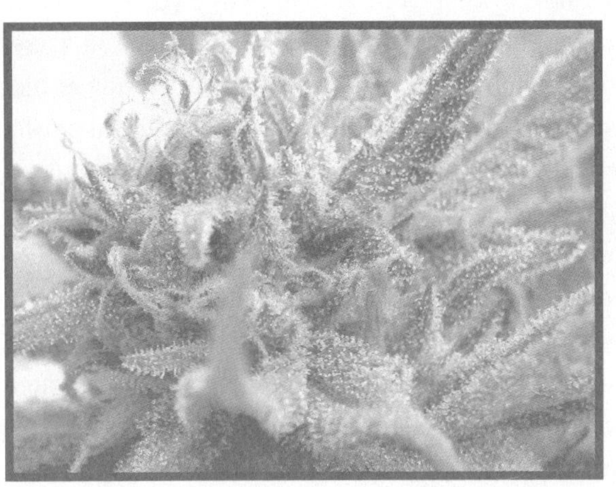

The tiny white crystals that cover the leaves and flowers are capitate-stalked resin glands

Cultivating those coveted THC crystals takes about four months. I'll guide you through the two main phases of cannabis cultivation: the vegetative stage (for growing leaves and stems) and the flowering stage (for growing buds). Every two months vegetative plants will move to the budding stage, budded plants will be harvested, and a new generation of plants will start the vegetative stage from vegetative plant clippings also called cuttings. This cycle ensures a regular supply of smokeable cannabis as long as you're willing to keep growing it.

Security

Before we get to growing your marijuana, let's consider how to keep your garden — and you — safe and secure. Pot gardens are often camouflaged in secret rooms. Some growers use trap doors or entrances hidden behind false walls. I heard of a commercial grower who buried railway cars to grow pot. Other grow operations are located on remote farms or properties far from civilization. All of these secret growing places have been busted. Why? The growers either sold their weed to someone and it was traced back to the source, or told someone about their operation. Forget about infrared detection and odor-sniffing surveillance dogs because most (probably 95 percent) of police busts are a result of good old-fashioned stool pigeons. Once people start bragging about their grow-ops, the elaborate subterfuge and alarm systems become useless. Some people even give guided tours of their pot farms to friends and acquaintances for no other reason than misguided pride in their gardening achievements. If you are not given to bragging, then all you need to grow pot is a private closet or room, preferably in the basement of your house.

You also need to be careful visiting hydroponics shops. If I were a cop and wanted to find out who was growing pot in the neighborhood, I would either set up an undercover sting operation in a local hydroponics store or start up my own. It would then be relatively simple to set up a surveillance team to follow a marijuana grower to his grow operation after he picks up a large load of supplies from the store. I'm certain this is done on occasion, and I always make clear to the salesperson that I have only a little indoor growing setup that I use for growing fresh herbs. If you are a commercial cannabis grower, it is wise to divide your purchase of supplies among several stores so as not to raise suspicions about the size of your garden. The only reason to visit a hydroponics shop when you are growing a container garden is for replacement indoor grow lamps and certain accessories such as pH meters and special timers. The less frequently you visit hydroponics stores, the better the security of your pot garden. When you do visit a hydroponics store, park your car some distance away and walk to the store. Always pay with cash. In general, you shouldn't chat with hydroponics and seed salespeople about anything to do with your pot growing other than the cost of equipment or the health of your "tomato plants." You might even suggest that the supplies you are buying are for someone else.

Paranoia is not a disease in the weed-growing business. It is good. It is necessary. Paranoia keeps you and your garden safe. It's not just the police you have to worry about these days. Rotten little thieves and even worse individuals with guns and bad attitudes will enter your home to steal your little bit of weed. Small operations are at a lesser risk because of the small payoff, but remember the Second World War slogan "Loose lips sink ships" and keep quiet about your garden. It's tempting to show off your results, but resist the temptation. If only *you* know about your garden, it will be safe.

For those of you into James Bond techniques, there are surveillance and monitoring systems available that will protect your grow room while you are absent. There are even systems to control nutrients and pH from remote locations, but they are very expensive and totally unnecessary for personal marijuana setups. If you want to go the commercial growing route, most hydroponics stores can obtain remote and automated systems for you.

How Many Plants Do I Need?

I recommend a simple container system for growing cannabis, which means your plants can be grown anywhere — in your living room, in a closet, or in a room of their own. If you're not sure where you'd like to grow, it may be helpful to consider how many plants you'll need. The average size of a full-grown indoor marijuana plant in bloom is about three to four feet tall. Each cannabis plant of that size, grown to maturity, will yield about two ounces of *dried* cannabis. (Note I said dried pot, not the shitty, wet stuff that street dealers often sell.) Each plant takes four months to grow from seed (or clone) to maturity. Therefore, each plant produces about two ounces of pot every four months. If you smoke an ounce of pot a week, you'll need a total of eight plants. Four plants will be growing in a vegetative state, and four plants will be growing in a budding state. The four plants in the vegetative state will produce nothing smokable, but the four plants in the budding state will produce two ounces of dried pot every two months, for a total of eight ounces. One ounce of primo dried pot per week is probably enough pot for most people who smoke bud and maybe even most couples. If you need less cannabis than that — say only a quarter of an ounce per week — you'll need only a quarter of the eight plants that a one-ounce-a-week smoker needs, a total of two plants — one in vegetative state and one in budding state.

Once you've decided how many plants you'll need, you can consider where you'd like to grow them and select one of the next three possibilities: growing weed around your house, growing in a closet or grow bag, or growing in a dedicated room (or rooms). I'll cover smaller setups first, and then we'll move on to the design of a custom grow room.

Smaller-Scale Growing

Just like regular house plants, a few cannabis plants can be scattered around a living room or dining room without any problems. The difference is that your house plants are in a perpetual state of dormancy, except for a brief growth spurt every spring. Your cannabis plants, on the other hand, are always kept in a vigorous growing state that requires a lot more watering and attention. During their flowering stage, they need at least 12 hours of undisturbed darkness every day for at least two months in order to bloom and produce buds. If you are growing cannabis in a living room, when the plants are budding you'll have to cover them with dark plastic for 12 hours a night because the television and house lights will prevent proper bud development. Don't just throw a plastic bag or cloth over them.

Build a wood or wire frame to keep the cloth or plastic covering from actually resting on the branches and "sweating" your plants, which can cause mold.

Use as much natural daylight as possible to grow your plants, and add lighting over their 12-hour light period on dark days and in winter months. You might have to turn on your supplemental lights early in the morning or evening when natural light is not strong enough to grow your plants. Supplemental lighting can be provided by LED lamps, 400-watt halide lamps, or even four banks of fluorescent grow lamps. Lamps of 1,000 watts are probably too bright and hot to use comfortably in a living room and are unnecessary for only a few plants.

Grow tents are practical tools for growing cannabis in an apartment or townhouse living area where there is no basement and only a few plants are required. These tents cost from one hundred to several hundred dollars, depending on size and features. They are flexible and mobile and solve the problem of creating a plastic night cover for your living room plants. Grow tents are self-contained with lighting, odor control, and vent fans suitable for cooling the small grow area. It is not a good idea to have other plants alongside your cannabis plants because any bugs on your house plants will eagerly jump or fly over to the cannabis plants, which generally provide a much tastier meal.

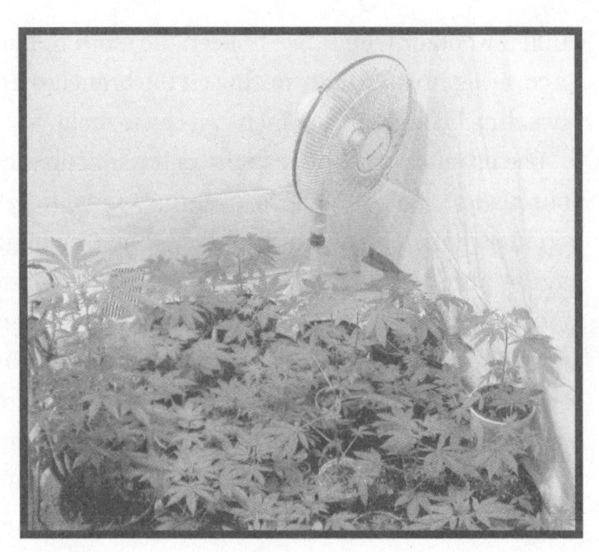

A grow tent in action

A walk-in closet can accommodate half a dozen plants or so as long as the closet is vented. A 400-watt metal halide lamp is a good fit for a closet grow-op. A 1,000-watt lamp is probably too hot. A 250-watt lamp can work but grows plants very slowly. You might try an LED grow light for vegetating cannabis, but a 400-watt light with a vented hood is probably the best all-around choice for both vegetating and budding cannabis in small spaces. The vegetative clones required for a closet grow-op should probably be grown in a different location, either in another closet or anywhere convenient, including under fluorescent lights beneath your ensuite bathroom counter.

Preparing Your Grow Room

Grow room walls should be painted white or covered with heavy duty white plastic or silver foil. A stapler is the best tool for attaching a foil or plastic wall covering unless the walls are concrete. With concrete walls, simply paint them white or nail 1"-wide wooden slats to the wall using concrete fasteners, and then staple the white plastic or silver foil to the slats. The plastic or foil can be purchased at any hydroponics store. If you intend to grow your cannabis in a spare room in the house that might be used in the future as living quarters, be sure to cover the walls with plastic to keep them clean and free of mildew while using the room to grow plants. Simply remove the plastic and repaint the walls if you decide to close down your grow room.

If you are growing pot in a basement with a concrete floor, just clean it and paint it white. It can be repainted gray or white or any color you prefer when you close down your pot-growing operation. If the floor is wood, put down a layer of heavy-duty plastic (available at hydroponics, hardware or carpet stores) over it. If you can't find one piece of plastic large enough, glue two or more pieces together and overlap them on the floor. Make sure the edges of the plastic are stapled a few inches above the floor at about baseboard height so that any water spills won't seep through the plastic onto the wood floor. As long as no water ever sits on the floor and stains it, a wood floor can be resanded and finished to look new whenever you want.

If you are growing pot on laminate wood floors or carpeted floors, put down a layer of plastic as previously indicated. Then, as if laying a floor, carefully place half-inch plywood panels over the plastic-covered carpet, cutting the plywood as necessary for a perfect fit. Use marine-grade plywood and fill any cracks or holes with wood filler. Fiberglass tape and resin can be used to seal the edges of the plywood to the wall and where two or more pieces of plywood butt together. When you have completed installation of the plywood, lay down another layer of heavy-duty plastic, making sure that the edges are stapled above the baseboard height. Growing pot on a carpeted floor is less than ideal, but it can be done.

I once saw an entire house (rented, of course) covered with wall-to-wall carpet, and the tenant was growing marijuana plants in every room. When it came time to close down the operation and move out, the plastic and plywood were removed from the walls and floors, and the carpets were shampooed and looked as good as new once the pile was vacuumed straight again.

Even with these precautions, you must be very careful with watering and moisture buildup. Use deep trays under your pots so that if you misjudge and overwater the plants, the trays will hold the overflow. Use a wet/dry shop vacuum to remove excess water from the plant trays and to immediately clean up any spills on the floors.

If there are windows in the grow room, they must be closed off so that your garden remains a secret from the outside world. A simple way to accomplish this privacy is to hang a pair of sheer curtains in the window and then screw a slightly larger plywood sheet (painted black on the window-facing surface) over the interior wall surrounding the window. This will block out all light from the grow room while presenting a normal appearance outside. If you want to get tricky, you can place a small lightbulb in the window that turns on and off by a timer to give the appearance of a lived-in room. If there is no other place to vent your room, a sliding window can be left open a few inches and a vent fan installed over a 5" hole cut into the plywood covering the window. But there are better ways of venting a grow room, which I'll explain later in detail.

Lighting Systems

Like the gasoline that makes a car go fast, light makes cannabis grow fast. The most common lighting systems for growing cannabis indoors are 1,000-watt metal halide and 1,000-watt high-pressure sodium lamps. The former is the best for vegetative growth, while the latter is best for bud growth when a plant is blooming. These are the most powerful lighting systems available, and for larger operations of eight plants or more they grow the best cannabis. For smaller areas, such as closets, a 400-watt metal halide or sodium system is preferred because it produces less heat in a confined space than a 1,000-watt system. A 1,000-watt lighting system is best suited to a 10' × 10' or larger room and requires more aggressive temperature control with vented lamp hoods, air conditioners, or swamp coolers. A 600-watt halide system is also available and is reported to perform well in both the budding and vegetative stages of plant growth. But 600 watts is a little high for closet use and little small for budding plants in a larger room, so I have never had the need to really try one out.

LED systems are emerging as the new generation of lighting systems. These lighting systems offer as much brightness as conventional halide or sodium systems in light spectrums that are perfect for plants but look purple to the naked eye. LED systems offer this bright light without the electrical draw and heat buildup of halide or sodium lamps. The main problem with LED lights today is cost. They are very expensive, at about three times the cost of equivalent halide or sodium systems. LED systems have been found to work well for vegetative growing, for which they are pretty much as effective as conventional systems. However, they do not compare favorably with halide or sodium lights when it comes to flowering plants. So forget about LEDs for plants in bloom — for now.

If you're budgeting for electricity use, in British Columbia the approximate electrical costs for running an indoor grow-room setup with one 1,000-watt hi-pressure sodium lighting system (for budding plants) and one 400-watt halide lighting system (for vegetating plants) including all related growing equipment (such as fans and pumps and timers, but not including a room air conditioner) is about $100 per month. These costs may vary depending on location and may increase with additional lights or equipment.

Lighting systems can be purchased from any hydroponics store and should include ballasts, lamps, ballast boxes, lamp hoods, and wall plugs. All lights should be hung on chains with S-hooks for adjusting the height of the lights up or down in the grow room, and lamps should be kept approximately 1' to 2' above the plants, although they can be a few inches closer when using vented hoods. Run electrical cords along the ceiling, supporting the cord with swag hooks. Ballasts should be raised off the ground on concrete blocks to prevent damage from accidental water spills, and should be enclosed in a vented metal ballast box for safety reasons. You don't need an electrician to assemble this system, as the entire lighting setup can be provided by the hydroponics store ready to go. All you have to do is hook the hooded lamp to a ceiling hook, place the ballast box on a concrete block, and plug the wall plug into an outlet or a heavy-duty timer.

If anything ever goes wrong with this system, check timers first, then try changing the lightbulbs. In fact, you should change your lightbulbs every six months without fail. If you don't change your bulbs every six months, your plants will grow more slowly and become wispy and unhealthy. Wait until a halide or high-pressure sodium lightbulb has cooled down before attempting to change it, and change all of your lightbulbs at the same time — that way you won't forget any. If changing the lightbulb doesn't solve your lighting problem, simply unplug the cord, unhook the light fixture from the ceiling hooks, and take the setup (ballast, wiring, lightbulb, and hood reflector) back to the hydroponics store or to a licensed electrician to be fixed. Do not open the ballast box or touch or prod it, for it is made to deliver high voltage.

Some growers use light movers, which are either tracked or rotating systems that move lights around the room. The idea is that a moving light system will cover more area since plants can take in only a certain amount of light per hour. The difference that light movers make is slight, and they are completely unnecessary for a small garden (under 10' × 10').

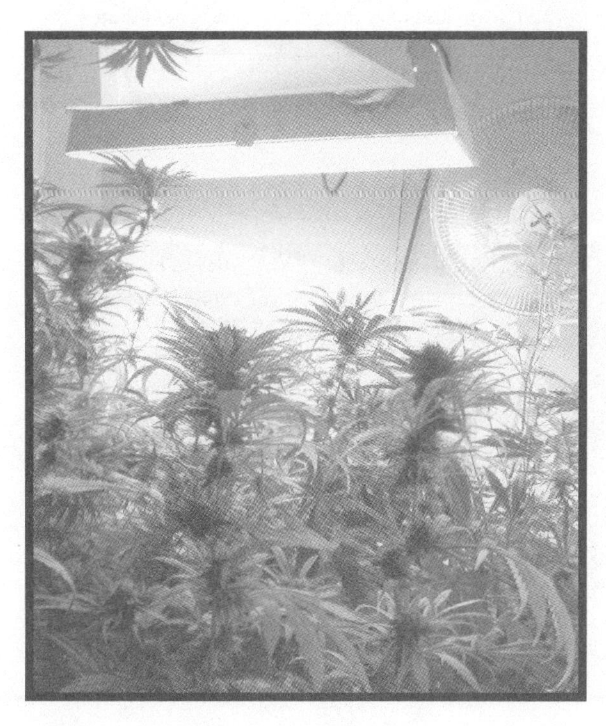

A high pressure sodium lighting system, with an exercise fan in the upper right corner

FIGURE 1: Choosing a Lighting System

Number of Plants	FEWER THAN 8	
Light	400-watt halide	400-watt sodium
Best for	Vegetative growth	Flowering growth
Pros	Generates less heat than a 1,000-watt halide	Generates less heat than a 1,000-watt sodium
Cons	Grows plants more slowly than a 1,000-watt halide	Grows plants more slowly than a 1,000-watt sodium
Approximate Cost	$200	$200

	UP TO 16	FROM 8 TO 16
1,000-watt halide	1,000-watt sodium	LED
Vegetative growth	Flowering growth	Vegetative growth
Best lamp available for growing vegetative plants	Best lamp available for growing buds	Comparable to halide lamps for growing vegetating plants but generates much less heat and requires much less electricity
Generates significant heat — lamps can burn flesh or explode if accidently broken or sprayed with cold water	Generates significant heat — lamps can burn flesh or explode if accidently broken or sprayed with cold water	Very expensive and there are lots of ineffective LED grow light systems
$300	$300	$500–$1,000 for top of the line LED systems such as the 90-watt UFO or 540-watt Mothership brand

Vent Fans

Vent fans remove both moisture and heat from the grow room and pull fresh air into the growing chamber. Vent fans are necessary whenever you are placing a large number of plants in a single room. A few plants (five or six) scattered around your house or living room won't need vent fans. But a lot of plants crammed into a small room will definitely need a fan that expels air through a dryer vent to a chimney, attic, or into another room.

The fan must be rated to remove a roomful of air every five minutes. The rating is shown on the box or on the fan itself. To calculate the volume of air in your grow room, multiply the height of the room by its width and length. For example, a 15' × 15' room with an 8' ceiling will have a room volume of 1,800 cubic feet (15 × 15 × 8 = 1,800). Therefore, a room fan for this room must be rated to remove 1,800 cubic feet of air within five minutes. Fans are rated in CFM (cubic feet per minute), so to calculate the CFM you need, divide the room volume by five. Therefore, a vent fan for an 1,800-cubic-foot room must be rated for at least 360 CFM. The fan can be rated higher, and the healthiest indoor gardens I have seen use massive vent fans, such as those employed by renovation companies to dry out water-damaged houses. These fans need larger openings than a standard 4" dryer vent and are often vented into attics or up chimneys.

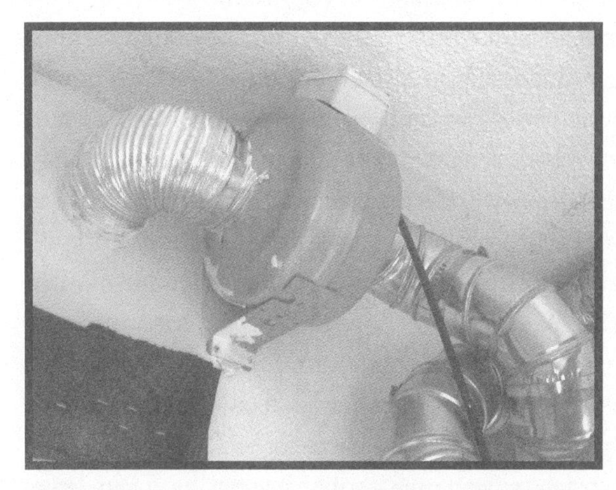

Installed vent fan

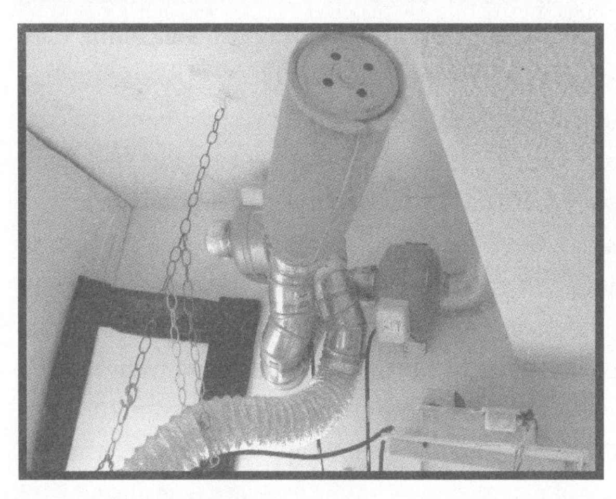

Charcoal air filter as part of a venting system

For fewer than 30 plants, the 4" centrifugal blower-style vent fans will suffice. They connect to dryer vents that run through the exterior walls. If a dryer vent is already in place and not being used, you can hook a length of 4" dryer vent hose between the vent and your grow room vent fan. If you need another dryer vent, they are easy to install. Rent a 4"-diameter hole saw at a tool rental shop (no way your home hand drill will do the job) and drill through your interior and exterior walls, making certain to avoid any 2" × 4" studs and electrical wires that might be running through the walls. For those of you who prefer not to do heavy work, hire a handyman to drill the hole for you. Then have him push a dryer vent tube, available at any hardware store, into the hole. The exterior end of the aluminum tube should have a flapper to prevent insects from entering, and the vent hose attaches to the interior end. To connect your vent fan to the dryer vent, use 4" vent pipes sold in hardware stores that connect together in sections rather than the polyester flexible vent hose with ridges along it. The ridges lessen the airflow and can create more noise than the metal pipe. It's not a big deal if you use the flexible hose, but if possible use the smooth metal type. Another method is to vent the grow room air up a fireplace chimney if there is one. Install a sheet of plywood to cover the fireplace opening and cut a hole (usually 4" to 5" in diameter) into the plywood for the vent fan. Do not vent your pot garden into a floor water drain since the odor ends up in the sewer system, where city workers can smell it and trace it back to you.

Ideally, your grow room should be vented outdoors. Try to position the vent as far away as possible from neighbors who might smell your plants. If you are growing more than half a dozen plants, you can buy a charcoal filter, which will remove or disguise any odor from your garden before it is vented outside. You can also use an ozone generator to remove odors from a room, but it can be harmful to plants and people.

Grow rooms can also be vented into a catch basin such as a garage, attic, chimney, or adjacent room if necessary. Most garages are not sealed against the weather, and vented odors will dissipate into the outside atmosphere through cracks, crevices, and the opening of the garage door. If you have a well-sealed garage, open a window or leave the garage door open an inch at the bottom. If you are venting into an adjacent room, find some way of venting the room to the outside or another room. The moisture from your grow room will dissipate easily and rapidly in a hallway or a room that has no plants in it. Unless you have a large grow operation with over 30 plants, moisture buildup will not be a problem.

Heat buildup is more of a problem in most small grow rooms. The ideal temperature for a grow room is between 70 and 80 degrees Fahrenheit. I like to keep my grow garden at about 78 degrees. You'll also need to monitor humidity, which should be at 50–60 percent for blooming plants and 60–70 percent for vegetative plants. (An electric thermometer/hygrometer, available for about $150 at hydroponics stores, will keep track of the high and low temperatures as well as the moisture levels in a grow room.) If venting fails to cool down your grow room to a maximum of 80 degrees Fahrenheit, you can use swamp coolers or preferably air conditioners to keep the room from overheating. Both will work but air conditioners cool better and also remove moisture whereas swamp coolers do not. Some stand-alone air conditioners work without venting kits and can just be placed in a room. The air conditioners I prefer have separate hoses for air intake and exhaust. They vent hot air from inside the room and draw cool air from outside the room and they don't send any odor out.

The last use for fans is to encourage sturdy growth. Exercise fans will keep your plants healthy and their branches firm and strong. Keep your exercise and vent fans running 24 hours a day unless you are supplementing with CO_2, in which case use a timer to turn the vent fans off when the CO_2 gas is turned on. I don't recommend the use of CO_2 in non-commercial gardens. The heat buildup in the room and the aggravation of lugging heavy CO_2 tanks around are not worth the gains.

Vented Lamp Hoods

You can use vented light shades (hoods) to cool down a grow room in addition to vent fans. These airtight hoods enclose the top and sides of the lamp in aluminum and the side beneath the lightbulb with glass. Vent hoods are an inexpensive and efficient way to remove heat from a grow room, and they protect growers from the powerful lights that can cause serious burns. If there is only one 1,000-watt halide or sodium lightbulb in your grow room, you might not require anything more than one vent fan. In the case of a two-lamp 1,000-watt lighting system in a typical 12' × 16' room, you'll need a vented hood for each lamp. The air inside the hood is vented through a 4" hose to anywhere outside the garden. A similar hose is positioned at the opposite side of the light hood and runs to another location outside the grow room, pulling fresh, cool air through the hood to cool the lamp. Because cooling air is drawn from outside of the grow room and runs through the sealed hooded lamp system, the exhaust has no odor. Very little heat escapes into the grow room from one of these vented lamp hoods, and you can actually touch the glass under the hood while the lamp is on without burning your hand.

If you don't have a vented hood, I strongly advise you to turn off your grow lights when working in your indoor garden to protect against skin burns and eye damage from exploding lightbulbs. An accidental spray of cold water on a hot grow lamp can easily explode the bulb and send glass shards flying through the air. Even with vented hoods, you should really use a 100-watt light in the grow room for everyday garden work. Although the grow lights should be turned off during regular garden maintenance, they should definitely be left on when you wish to check your plants for insect damage. Such damage is much easier to see under the bright grow lights. If there are pests in your room, they often end up dead in a little pile lying on the glass inside your hooded grow lights. The evidence of these dead pests is often the first sign of an infestation.

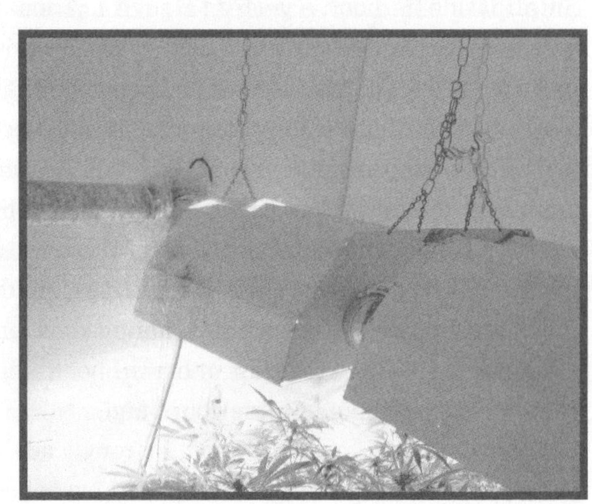

Vented hood lamps can be run in series

There is a slight loss of brightness while using hood vents because the light has to pass through the glass before contacting the plants. However, I strongly suggest that you use a vented hood system. The safety and convenience of hood vents are worth any minimal loss in lamp brightness.

Air Purifiers

When odor is a problem, you can use an ozone generator (a small appliance available at a hydroponics store) or air purifiers, available in many varieties with more innovative designs arriving on store shelves every day. Your local hydroponics store is the place to start researching the latest and greatest in odor control. The Internet is also a great resource for finding new products.

A simple yet effective way to manage odors in a grow room is with a vented collection chamber and an ozone generator. The collection chamber can be made using a 30-gallon garbage can. To make this DIY air purifier, **you'll need:**

- ☐ plastic or rubber 30-gallon garbage can with a lid
- ☐ jigsaw or bladed cutting device
- ☐ 4" flexible dryer hose (long enough to reach from your chamber to your vent exit hole)
- ☐ ozone generator

- ☐ duct tape
- ☐ picture hanging wire
- ☐ 2" swag hooks

Then follow these simple steps:

1. Cut a 4" hole in the center of the bottom of the garbage can.
2. Screw the garbage can lid in place and cut a similar 4" hole in the lid.
3. Push a 4" flexible dryer hose into the hole in the bottom of the garbage can.
4. Attach the other end of the hose to a vent fan that pushes air through the 4" diameter exit hole in your grow room.
5. Use duct tape to attach vent ducting and to seal venting system connections.
6. Hang the garbage can horizontally near the ceiling using wires and swag hooks.
7. Insert an ozone generator through the 4" opening in the garbage can lid.
8. Plug the appliance in.

The collection chamber will vent the warm air at the top of the room and mix it with the ozone. The vented air will now smell of ozone, not skunk weed, and neighbors won't be alerted to the aromas of your grow room. Because ozone generators are harmful to plants (and humans), it is best to vent the exhaust outside of the house and keep the vent fan attached to the collection chamber running at all times. If the vent fan stops working, ozonated air will flow out of the chamber and damage the plants.

A charcoal filter can also be used to combat exhaust odor. Attach the charcoal filter to the ceiling with wire and swag hooks and connect it with 4" dryer hose to a vent fan that pushes air out through a 4" hole in the grow-room wall. Charcoal filters are totally safe for both people and plants and are highly effective in removing odors. Replace your charcoal air filter once a year.

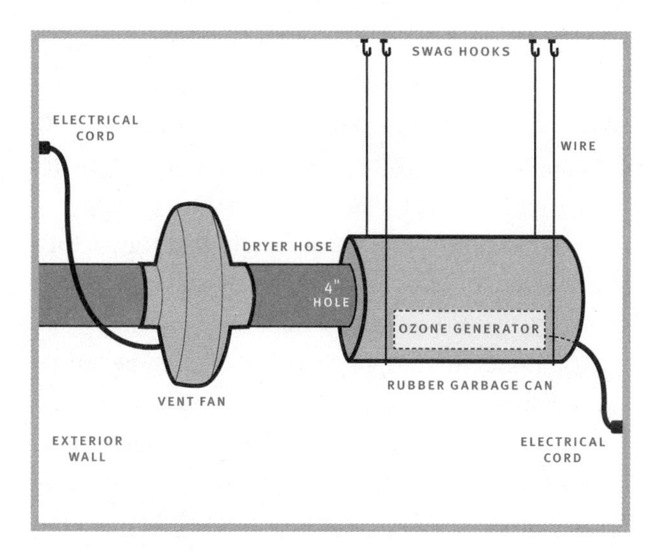

Timers

The lamps in your budding room should be turned on every day for 12 hours and then turned off for 12 hours. This is done simply with a 24-hour timer (available for about $25 at hardware or hydroponics stores). Set your timer so the lights are on during the time period you most want to work in your grow room. Outside the room, it can be day or night. As far as the plants are concerned, when the lights are off it is night, and when the lights are on it is day. Do not turn on any other light during the budding room's 12-hour periods of darkness because doing so might trigger the budding plants to return to a vegetative state. (I have made this mistake several times, and my budding plants did not revert to vegetative growth, but it can and will happen if a small light is left on for days or weeks during the budding room's 12-hour dark period.) If you accidently leave your budding lights on too long for any length of time up to a week, just make certain that they return to a regimen of 12-hour dark periods and your plants should suffer no permanent damage.

The lights in your vegetative room can be left on for 24 hours day after day without need of a timer. If you find that the lights in the vegetative room are generating too much heat, set a timer so the lights are on for 18 hours and off for six hours during every 24-hour period. That will allow the room to cool down somewhat for at least six hours every day without affecting the plant's growth and internal clock. Usually, the lights in the vegetative room are 400-watt halides that run a bit cooler than the 1,000-watt lights in the budding room, but since the vegetative room is often smaller it can still get quite hot.

Timers for both the 400-watt and the 1,000-watt halide and sodium lamps must be heavy-duty models and should be rated for at least 1,200 watts of power draw. Hydroponics stores will sell you the right type of timer, but if you decide to purchase a timer at a hardware store, pick one rated for 1,200 watts or better. If ever you experience a problem with the lighting system (lights that won't turn on or lights that turn on sooner or later than they should), check the timer first. As they age, timers sometimes burn out and either fail completely or start to run slow. If you see evidence of blackening, burning, or soot where the timer plugs into the wall outlet or at the connections where the light system plugs into the timer, throw it out and buy a new one. Same thing if it becomes noisy or starts to feel warm to the touch. Plan to replace a timer every few years or so.

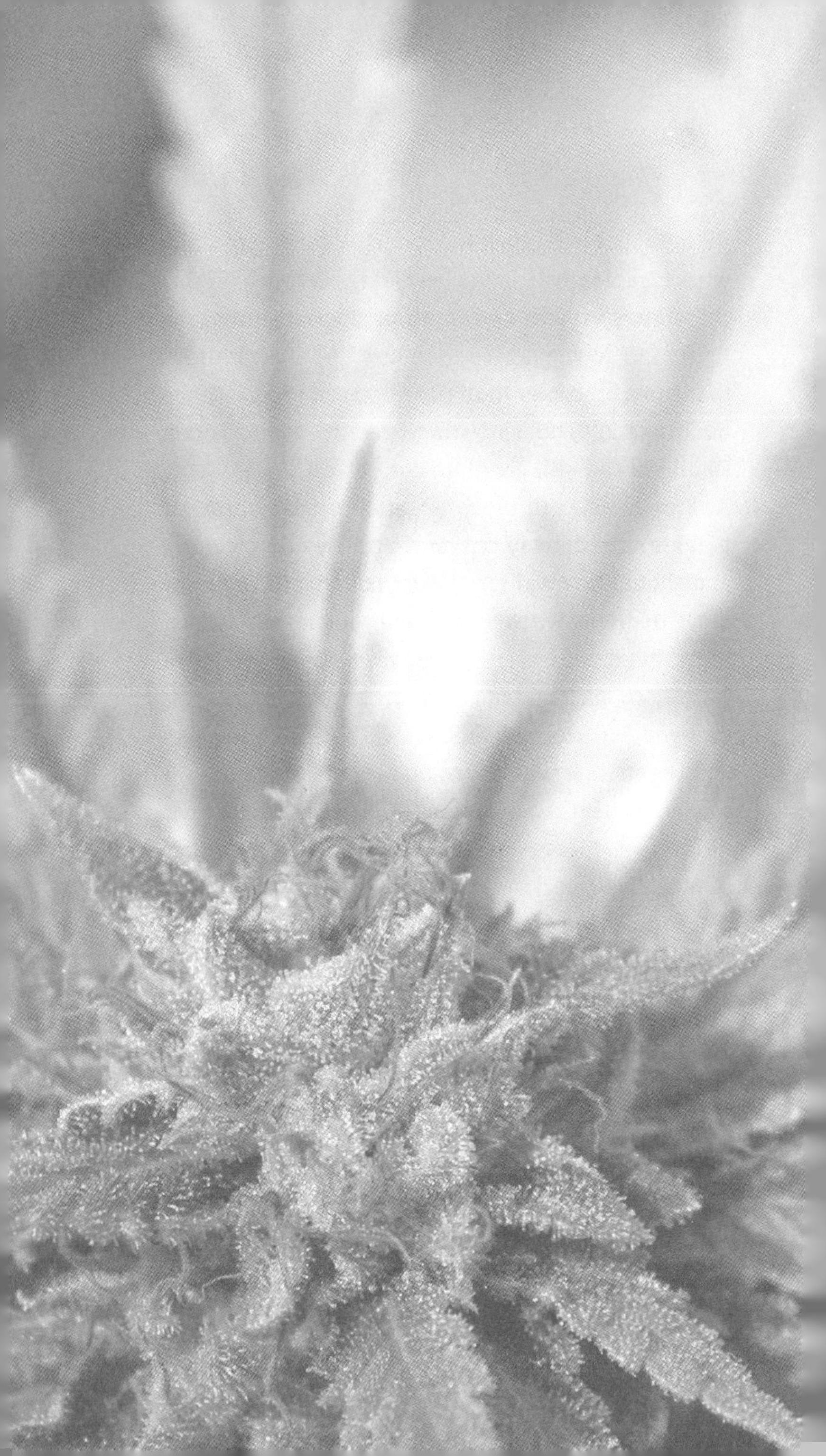

2

GROWING FUNDAMENTALS

Basic Gardening Supplies

A container system utilizes supplies available from any garden shop. I prefer five-gallon containers for my flowering weed and one-gallon containers for my vegetative weed. These containers can be found at most hardware stores and are less expensive than dedicated plant pots. The five-gallon pails allow for adequate root development and also come with convenient wire handles that fold down against the side of the container when not in use. Drill a series of quarter-inch holes at the bottom of the plant containers for drainage. If you make the holes any wider than that, your drainage stones will roll out. Containers can be white or black. Black is good for root development, while white is better at reflecting light away from the pots so that heat does not build up in the containers. If your room is air-conditioned, heat buildup won't be an issue. I prefer black pots and an air-conditioned grow room. Place plastic trays under every plant pot. Use the deepest trays you can find to prevent water from overflowing onto the floor. Some plastic buckets come with lids that are deep enough to use as trays.

You'll also need a water drum in your grow room. A 30-gallon plastic tank/garbage container holds just the right amount of water for gardens of up to 15 budding plants and 15 to 18 clones. Plastic garbage cans are available at any hardware store. Also pick up a fish tank bubbler to introduce air into the standing water. The bubbler can be purchased at either hydroponics or pet stores. Just drop it into the tank and plug it in. The bubbler runs all the time and does not require a timer.

For starting seeds and clones, I prefer using soil instead of soilless mix because there is enough nutrition in the soil for at least a month, and it is available to the plants with no danger of overfeeding or burning them with too much fertilizer. The best soil comes from hydroponics or gardening stores, but you can also use a brand-name product such as Miracle-Gro soil, which will have all of the necessary trace elements as well as nitrogen, phosphorous, and potassium in the soil. When you find a good soil stick with it.

Always use sterilized soil for your indoor garden to avoid bringing in pests and diseases. When your crop is harvested or your clones are transplanted, do not reuse the leftover soil or drainage rocks. Dump the soil and rocks into a garbage bag and buy fresh soil and drainage rock for the next crop. Toss the garbage bag into a local dumpster, making certain to remove all leaves and branches that might identify the garbage as pot. Place any pot leaves and branches in paper bags, and after they have dried, burn them in your fireplace if you have one. If you don't have a fireplace, save the leaf debris until you have enough to fill a garbage bag, and dispose of it any way you can. Burn it or bury it or scatter it in the woods. If you burn it, pick a time and place when the fewest people will be around to notice how good it smells.

For growing cannabis in the budding phase, I prefer soilless mediums such as Pro-Mix because it is sterile, light, and clean to use, and it drains well in plant pots. Soilless mixes are often closer than soil to the optimal pH of 7. Regular soil is very messy when wet and is hard to clean up compared with soilless mixes, which don't leave sludge behind after a wet cleanup. I like to use soilless mixes for blooming plants because I can "push" the plants with a large amount of fertilizer (when necessary) and then clear out the fertilizer with water that drains quickly. Use the most porous soil mix available, and in the case of Pro-Mix use the brand labeled "High Porosity." The soil substitute mixes are often in large bags that weigh about 30 pounds, but smaller half-size soil mixes are also available. You'll also need to buy lava rock or sterilized gravel for drainage at the bottom of each pot.

You'll need two types of fertilizer to bolster plant growth, one for each growth stage: bloom fertilizer to encourage big, healthy buds, and *vegetative* fertilizer to sponsor healthy growth going into the bud stage. Liquid fertilizers are more expensive, but I prefer them because they mix better than powdered fertilizers. I prefer Heavy Harvest by Nutrilife, but I have also used General Hydroponics plant food. When you find a good fertilizer, keep using it, because once you learn the mixing ratio it is easy to follow. Most good fertilizers contain a few trace elements (micronutrients) in addition to the basic ingredients of N, P, and K. If you buy premium plant food, as opposed to the cheapest plant foods, you'll get trace elements in a proper ratio to the basic elements. Vegetative plant food formulas are usually higher in nitrogen while flowering formulas are higher in potassium. I don't recommend the use of "bloom boosters" and "bud blasters" or any of the miracle growth aids sold in garden shops and hydroponics stores with the promise of increased plant yields. Invariably, these growth aids just add to the fertilizers you are already using and toxify the plant with too much of a good thing. When preparing a fertilizer solution use the mixing directions on the package as a guide, but use your salts meter to determine the precise ratio of fertilizer to water. (I'll cover more on fertilizing in chapter 3.)

Starting from Seed

A successful marijuana garden starts with good seeds. They can be purchased in Canada at retail outlets, by mail order, or over the Internet. To find the necessary seeds, look up "cannabis seeds" on the Internet and watch the search results pour in. If you order seeds by mail, do not have them sent to where your pot will be grown. Have them sent to a friend, relative, or mail drop address. In some parts of Canada (certainly in major cities) you can find walk-in retail stores that sell seeds.

It is still illegal under U.S. federal law to grow or possess marijuana or to sell seeds. Some states have overruled the federal marijuana laws on possessing and selling marijuana but marijuana seeds are still a gray legal area. Although some U.S. cannabis dispenseries are reported to sell cannabis seeds, they are not generally allowed to be sold in the U.S. at this time. So to obtain seeds in America you will have to shop around a little harder than in Canada. You can try asking about seeds at your local medical marijuana compassion clubs or cannabis dispensaries. (Do not expect positive results over the phone.) Often the attendant there can direct you to someone that can help you even if they are unable to sell you the seeds themselves. Cannabis magazines like *High Times* or *Cannabis Culture* have advertisements for mail order seeds, and online sites may offer to mail cannabis seeds into the U.S., or you could try to find seeds or clones from a contact in the weed-growing underworld. Your local hydroponics shops can probably direct you to someone with seeds or clones if they don't think you're a narc. Your pot supplier can be the greatest help of all in finding a seed or clone source, although he will ultimately be disappointed to lose your business. Whatever your plan, I do not advise carrying seeds in your clothing or luggage or anywhere on your person when traveling through immigration or customs in any country.

Do not take seeds from a bag of pot you purchased to start your garden. These seeds are often hermaphrodites that grow unwanted male parts along with the desired female parts and are guaranteed to give you the same or worse "seedy bush" weed as the bag that they came from. Seeds from purchased weed might also be from an outdoor variety that does not grow well indoors. What you want for your indoor marijuana garden is a hybrid Sinsemilla plant. *Sinsemilla*, a Spanish word, means "without seeds." Seeds can take up half of your marijuana crop and thereby reduce your return by 50 percent. They lower the potency of your pot, and seed pods make the pot taste bitter. The best seeds are large and waxy, though all cannabis seeds will produce marijuana. Visit your local seed store or website to select the seeds that best suit your requirements and tastes.

When you have secured your seeds and are ready to start the growing process, **gather:**

- ☐ saucer
- ☐ cotton balls or paper towels
- ☐ sterilized potting soil
- ☐ potting containers
- ☐ pencil

Then,

1. Place seeds on a saucer in thoroughly moistened cotton balls or paper towels for several days until a white root comes out. Keep the cotton balls or paper towels thoroughly moist but not soaked, adding water daily if necessary.
2. Fill one-gallon containers with soil-based growing medium or seed-starting soil.
3. Water soil.
4. Using a pencil-sized object, poke a hole about a half inch deep in the soil.
5. Place the seed in the hole with the root facing down.
6. Gently fill in the gaps around the seeds with loose soil and continue to add soil until the seeds are completely covered with a thin layer of dirt.
7. Let the seeds germinate in darkness or low light, waiting until they sprout before placing them under full light.

Water seedlings daily if necessary to keep the soil damp. Only wet the top inch or so of soil but do not let the soil medium dry out. Use a spray bottle type to mist the seedlings when they sprout to prevent water from knocking over the tender plants. If the seedlings do fall over, don't lift them up or stake them upright. They will stand again on their own after a few days of lying down.

After a month or so, when the soil-borne nutrition is all used up by the growing plants, begin adding fertilizer at about half strength. I feed my vegetating plants about every two weeks. For more information on fertilizing, see chapter 3.

Determining Sex

After one to two months of vegetative growth, when cannabis plants are about 1' tall, they can be placed in the budding room under 12 hours of light per day. Within two weeks the male flower pods first appear at the trunk of the male plants, usually where a branch is growing. A female plant will show similar shaped flower pods on the main stem but these flower pods quickly develop white pistils (hairs) that do not appear on males. The 1 mm to 2 mm round flower pods of male plants will sometimes resemble a female flower for a brief time, showing two protruding spear-shaped leaves that look like flower pistils, but by the time they are one month old, none of the male seed pods show clusters of white pistils like female flowers do. If left unattended the male plants will form clusters of tiny white or yellow flowers that eventually release a pollen that fertilizes the white female flower pistils to create seeds and propagate the species. When that happens the female plant spends all of its energy producing seeds and produces very little smokable bud. To avoid the complications of sexing your plants, you can sometimes buy feminized seeds that are the result of fertilizing a female plant with a hermaphrodite male. The resultant seeds from a feminized plant are purely female but are not reliable for breeding because of their tendency to produce hermaphrodites. For more on breeding, see chapter 4.

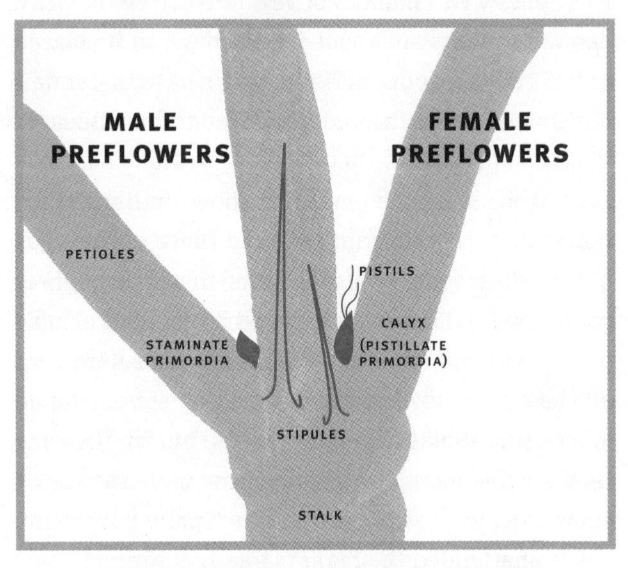

Female flowers develop clusters of white pistils (hairs) that protrude from their seed pods

Cloning Plants

The simplest way to start your garden is with cannabis seeds, but once your garden is under way, plant clones are essential to keep your marijuana garden rotating from crop to crop with the least amount of cost and effort. Here is a step-by-step method for cloning. It is simple and consistent. **You'll need:**

- ☐ sterilized soil
- ☐ one-gallon plastic or clay plant containers (about 8" wide and 8" deep)
- ☐ bottle of Rootone or equivalent root growth stimulant
- ☐ sterilized razor blade

To start cloning,

1. Prepare containers by filling them with soil.
2. Select a cutting. You want a healthy piece, not some scraggly piece. Slice it off at a 45 degree angle with a razor blade.
3. Remove the leaves and small side branches from the base of the cutting using the razor blade, leaving a nice cluster of leaves at the top of the cut.
4. Dip the cut end in rooting solution and shake off the excess powder or gel.

5. Make a hole in the prepared soil; make the hole wider than the plant's stem so the rooting hormone won't be scraped off.
6. Place the cutting into the hole and gently pack the medium around it.
7. Using plain water, soak the cuttings in the soil.
8. Place cuttings under low light until roots develop.

There's really no need to prepare extra clones for insurance, as I find that well over 98 percent of my healthy cuttings survive the cloning process.

Basic Care During Vegetative Growth

Vegetative growth is the time prior to flowering when a plant grows its leaves and branches. This phase lasts approximately two months and requires 18 to 24 hours of light per day. A healthy vegetating plant will be dark green. The stems will be thick, and the plant will stand upright in a typical Christmas tree shape. The branches will be rubbery and strong, and the leaves will not tear easily.

Cuttings do not require plant food/fertilizer until their roots develop about three to four weeks after being planted, and you should use a weak mix for the first feeding. I never exceed a reading of 8 on my salts meter when mixing fertilizer for my young cuttings. If the young plants react well to the fertilizer, keep feeding them approximately every two weeks. You'll have to determine what the best schedule is for your own plants, which might be different from mine based on your growing climate, the porosity of the soil mix, and the vigor of the cannabis strain you choose. Choose a fertilizer high in nitrogen, also known as vegetative formula, for this phase of leafy growth.

A vegetating plant does not mind if you turn the lights off for a few hours. As long as there are at least 18 hours of light per session, the plant will experience vigorous growth. If lights are accidentally left off for a few hours or even days, there is no lasting harm to a vegetating cannabis plant. If heat buildup becomes a problem in the grow room during vegetative plant growth, turn the lights off for six hours per day and begin an 18-hour-per-day growth regimen that will allow the room to cool down during the off-light cycle. Don't worry about triggering your vegetating plants into budding when turning the light cycle down to 18-hour days. It takes at least two weeks of 12 hours of light per day to trigger a vegetative plant into blooming.

Water vegetative plants twice a week or more often if needed with pure water from your water container. Let tap water stand in the container for a day before using it to water the plants. This will allow the chlorine in the water to evaporate. Chlorinated tap water won't really hurt your plants, but it is better to let the chlorine escape and to let the water reach room temperature before using it on the plants. Very cold water can shock the plant and stunt growth.

Trimming during the vegetative state is good for making bushy plants, but *never* trim a plant once it is budding and in flower. When your plants have reached the end of their vegetative growth period, take a cutting from each plant before transplanting it and moving it to the budding room. This keeps your garden stocked with new plants as needed.

Transplanting Seedlings and Clones

When the cuttings or seedlings have completed the vegetative stage and are about two months old and two feet tall, they are ready to be transplanted and moved to the budding room. **You'll need:**

- ☐ five-gallon planting containers with ¼" drainage holes in the bottom.
- ☐ lava rock or commercially sterilized gravel
- ☐ Pro-Mix or another commercial growing medium, preferably soilless
- ☐ water or a mild quarter-strength bloom fertilizer formula

After you have the materials,

1. Prepare the receptor plant pot so that it is half full of soilless mix.
2. Position your donor plant pot directly over the receptor plant pot.
3. Place a finger on either side of the seedling or clone's main stem and turn the donor pot upside down. The seedling or clone should easily slip out into your hand. If the donor plant does not easily slip out of a plastic pot, squeeze all around the pot to break the seal of the soil against the sides of the container and then try again. For a clay pot turn it upside down and tap the sides and bottom with a rubber mallet until the donor plant slides out into your palm or receptor pot.
4. Flip your palm over and place the seedling or clone and its root ball into the receptor pot.
5. Add soil or mix around the root ball until it fills the receptor pot to a couple of inches below the top.
6. Water the plant to settle the soil around the roots, using pure water or a mild quarter-strength bloom fertilizer formula.
7. Move the transplanted seedling or clone to the budding room.

Basic Care During Flowering Growth

Flowering growth lasts about two months and follows two months of vegetative growth. Some cannabis plants require two and a half or three months of flowering to reach maturity, while others can shave a few days off the two-month flowering time and be ready after six or seven weeks of flowering. It all depends on the genetics of the plant you choose to grow.

Flowering growth requires 12 hours of light per day followed by 12 hours of uninterrupted darkness. Even a small light left on during the 12-hour night period can stop a plant from flowering and send it back into its vegetative cycle. Fertilizers that have a lot of potassium are essential in this part of the plant's development. Most of the heavy bud growth occurs during the final two weeks of blooming, and if you harvest even a week or two early you'll get skimpy buds that are half the weight and half the flavor of a fully developed bud. If you run out of smoke near the end of the budding cycle it is better to buy some weed than cut down your budding plants a week or two early.

Plants in bud stretch during the first few weeks of the 12-hour light regimen, sometimes growing twice as tall as they started before they are finally harvested. Once plants are over three feet tall, support them by tying them to bamboo stakes. If a plant grows too tall during its blooming cycle and comes too close to the lamps, bend it, don't trim it. Squeeze the stalk at the bend and slowly force it so that it is horizontal to the floor, being careful not to snap the branch off. Once the plant is bent, leave it alone to recover — which it will. Trimming a budding plant stops any further growth along the limb. If you must trim a budding plant for any reason, trim a side branch but not the main stem. Trimming the main stem will stop or slow growth in the entire plant, while trimming a branch stops growth only in that branch. So, if you must try a sample of your weed, cut a branch, not the trunk.

When feeding your plants during flowering growth, keep an eye on the white flowering tips. If the pistils (white hairs) of the flowers begin to turn brown within a few days of feeding, it is an obvious sign of overfertilizing. Too much water or fertilizer and most insecticides will cause the white pistils to turn brown. Cannabis plants are very sensitive during flowering and should be monitored closely.

CO_2 Injection

I don't recommend CO_2 injection for personal growers due to the constant exposure to hydroponics stores for CO_2 tank refills. CO_2 injection is a needless expense. It might increase the yield slightly, but it also requires closing the vent fans in your room, which leads to heat buildup that damages your plants. Having stated all these negatives, though, a properly set-up CO_2 injection system can encourage vigorous growth and promote bushy plants that grow to maturity about a week faster than normal.

Hydroponics

You might hear a lot about hydroponics as being the best way of growing indoors these days. It is not. The same is true of aeroponics and flood and drain systems. The problem with all of these hydroponics systems is that they pump water and nutrients into the plants, and then the water returns to a common tank to be used again. That means all the plants share the same used water, so any water-borne viruses, diseases, or bacteria are shared by all plants. If one plant happens to pick up a bad infection, it will spread like wildfire through the entire garden.

My hydroponics garden once contracted a case of rust, and it spread to every plant. I had to start my garden over again from seeds. Similarly, root rot spread through my hydroponics garden one time, and it wiped out my plant crop and continued to infect my future plants even though I sterilized the entire garden, pots, lines, and pumps. I scrubbed walls and floors with bleach. I changed to a whole new strain of plants. And still the plants in my garden developed slimy root rot and died. I realized then I'd have to throw everything away and start with all new seeds, pots, and equipment. That is when I decided not to take a chance with hydroponics ever again, even though I had several decades of success using such growing methods. I went back to individual container growing, in which excess water and nutrients evaporate instead of returning to a common water trough, and I never had root rot or rust problems again. If one of my plants did happen to contract a disease, I could simply remove it from the garden without contaminating all the other plants.

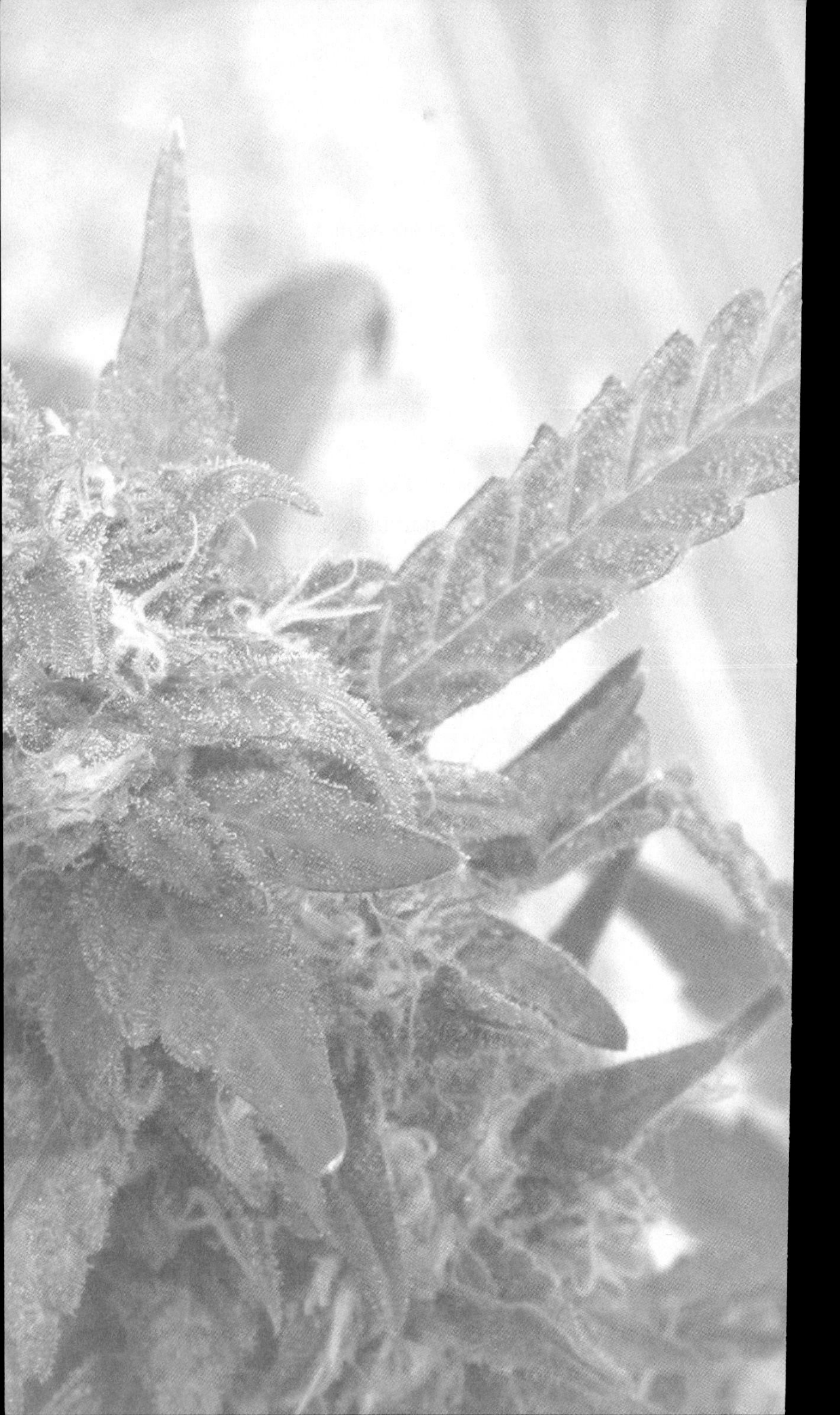

3

MAINTAINING *your* GARDEN

With beginner's luck and a modicum of knowledge about growing plants, it is possible to grow a bumper crop of pot even on your first try. The trick is to produce a heavy harvest of pot on successive tries. One reason that might explain why beginners often grow a good first crop is a result of hybrid vigor. Most commercial cannabis seeds today are crossbreeds or hybrids that for the first crop grow stronger and heartier than the second generation plants will, and in subsequent crops clones will become successively weaker. But clones are so much cheaper and easier to deal with than starting from seeds that the advantages of cloning exceed the drawbacks. In order to compensate for the weakening of the plants over time it is imperative to take advantage of every trick in this book. It is tempting to take shortcuts, but avoid the temptation. Every little detail I have included is for a good reason. Now let's get started.

pH Levels

Healthy plants are grown in soil or soilless mix with a pH level of around 7, which can be measured on a pH pen/meter (available from hydroponics stores for around $100). Such a pen is invaluable in growing plants indoors and allows you to monitor pH levels in both soil and water. Be sure to check the units of measure on the brand of pen you are using, as they may vary.

Check the pH of your water reservoir on a regular basis and keep it as close to pH 7 as you can. You can use pH up or pH down solutions (available at hydroponics stores) to balance your water to a reading of 7. Try not to put too much pH adjuster in the water at any one time. If you mess up and put in too much pH up, don't put in pH down to rebalance the water. Better to drain your water and start over with clean water. Having a perfect pH of 7 isn't useful if your solution has too many chemicals and not enough pure water. If after adding fertilizer to your water reservoir, you add pH up and then find that your final pH reading is 5.8 instead of 6.3 to 7 (the perfect range for pH) just leave things alone and go with that. If you try rebalancing with too much pH up or pH down, you may find your salts and pH meter readings are bouncing up and down and they may be unable to accurately read the final mix.

Ideally you must try to feed your plants a fertilizer and water mix that has been perfectly balanced to a pH of 6.3 to 7. Adding fertilizer to water will lower the pH of the water, so you'll probably need to adjust it with a little pH up. Once you become familiar with the amounts of fertilizer and pH up required for your garden, start adding pH up before you add fertilizer. You will require less pH up if you add it before the fertilizer. It may require a little practice to become familiar with the levels of pH up and fertilizer required, but in time it will become second nature. A monthly check with a soil slurry will show a reading of the pH that has built up in your soil or soilless medium. Read further along this chapter for more information on how to conduct a soil slurry test.

Salts Levels

Salts levels indicate the strength of fertilizers and can be determined using an EC pen, also known as a salts meter, invaluable in growing healthy marijuana and at $100, a worthwhile purchase from the hydroponics store. EC or electrical conductivity indicates how much dissolved salt is in a given sample. That is why EC is also referred to as TDS (Total Dissolved Salts) or Salinity (the amount of salts in a solution). All nutrients are salts, so EC is the same as measuring total nutrients in a solution. The water in your reservoir should have no salts in it and thus show a 0 reading on your salts pen when tested. When fertilizer is correctly proportioned into the water reservoir your salts pen should show a reading no higher than 10 for budding plants (8 is ideal) or 14 for vegetative plants (12 is ideal). If you goof up your fertilizer mix and end up with too much fertilizer, add water to bring the salts/fertilizer level down or change the water and start over. If a slurry of one part water and one part soil tests above 5 on the salts pen, it means the plants are getting too much fertilizer. If it tests below 3, the plants are getting too little fertilizer. A slurry reading of 4 on the salts pen is perfect.

Feeding

Ever wonder why some weed is bitter and goes out all the time between puffs? The answer, in a nutshell, is fertilizer. Too much fertilizer will ruin your weed. How much and how often you feed your plants are perhaps the trickiest parts for novice growers. As I've mentioned, every two weeks is a good feeding schedule for indoor vegetating plants and every three weeks for indoor flowering plants.

Before testing your water pH and fertilizer levels, test your pH and salts meters for accuracy using a test solution (available at any hydroponics shop). Simply dunk your pH meter in a small glass of the pH 7 test solution and check the reading. If adjustment is needed, turn the adjustment screw on the meter until the readout number on the pen reads 7. Then you can test the pH of your water. The same goes for testing your salts meter. The correct salts test solution registers 10 on the meter. By adjusting the set screw, you can adjust your salts meter until it reads a perfect 10 in the test solution. The salts meter is much more reliable than the pH meter and keeps its settings longer between adjustments, but I still check it almost every time I use it. After testing or using your meters rinse them off in clean water before putting them away.

You are not supposed to reuse the salts and pH test solutions in case they have become contaminated. I make certain to change my testing solutions once a year.

It takes some practice to get the amount of fertilizer right, but it helps to do your experimenting outside of your water reservoir until you calculate the appropriate amounts.

I follow a simple procedure I recommend for anyone starting out. **You'll need:**

- ☐ two-gallon bucket
- ☐ teaspoon
- ☐ tablespoon
- ☐ measuring cup
- ☐ two-part fertilizer formula
- ☐ salts meter
- ☐ pH meter

Then follow these steps:

1. Fill a two-gallon bucket with water from your reservoir.
2. Add one to two teaspoons of pH up and stir the water.
3. Following the directions on the label, add about three tablespoons of part one of the nutrient formula and stir.
4. Following the directions on the label, pour another three tablespoons of part two of the nutrient formula and stir.

5 Check the salts level with your salts pen. It should be between 10 and 12 parts per 1,000 (ppt), which will show as 10 or 12 on your salts meter.

6 Measure the solution in the bucket with a pH meter. The pH should be between 6.3 and 7.0 on your pH meter. If either of these numbers is not reached, simply increase the amounts of pH up and/or fertilizer until the proper numbers are obtained, keeping track of the amounts. If pH readings in your test bucket are too high, do not add pH down to the water. Simply empty the bucket and start over with a fresh two gallons of water and put in less pH up to start.

7 Once you reach the appropriate pH and salts levels, calculate how many two-gallon buckets are in your water reservoir. (In a 30-gallon reservoir, it would be 15.) Then multiply your two-gallon pH and fertilizer measurements by that number, and use a measuring cup to add the appropriate amounts of pH up and/or fertilizer to your water reservoir. Remember to always add the pH up ahead of your nutrients.

Do not expect to use the same water to fertilizer ratios when mixing bloom fertilizer as you do when mixing vegetative formula. Each fertilizer requires its own mixing ratios. After a few tries, it becomes relatively easy to get a perfect mixture of pH and nutrients.

If your fertilizer ratios are off, your plants will tell you. An unhealthy or overfertilized cannabis plant will look yellow and weak, often drooping its branches, and it might show signs of burning on the edges of its leaves, which can become reddish brown and dead looking. When a cannabis plant is seriously burned by overfertilizing, its leaves might become pock marked with dead patches. Underfeeding is sometimes indicated by red stems and branches, but when cannabis leaves turn red it is usually a genetic trait and not a sign of distress.

If your plants show any of these symptoms, or after several feedings you should test the pH and fertilizer/salts levels of the soil in your plant pots by making a soil slurry. Think of the soil slurry as a thermometer that measures the health of your plants. To make a slurry you mix one part of pH 7 room temperature water and one part soil until the soil has the consistency of molasses. Take the soil sample from the rootball of the plant rather than the surface of the plant pot, and don't worry about tearing a few root hairs out in the process. Let the solution stand for several minutes; then strain the mix through a coffee filter and place your salts meter into the slurry to take a reading. If your salts reading is 4–6, your soil has the perfect amount of fertilizer.

If the salts reading is too high (above 8), rinse the plant soil with several gallons of water, and wait at least two weeks before testing with a soil slurry again. Keep testing every two weeks and do not begin fertilizing again until the salts readings drop to between 4 and 6 in your slurry test. You might want to use a clearing agent like General Hydroponics FloraKleen, which will dissolve away accumulated fertilizer as it releases the nutrient bond between plants and salts. The clearing agent can also be used in the final flush of your plants one week before harvest to wash away the bitter taste from heavily fertilized weed

If the salts reading is too low (below 3) in your initial slurry test, increase the frequency of fertilizing without exceeding the strength of the fertilizer and water mix beyond 8 on the salts meter for flowering plants or 12 for vegetating plants. After several feedings under the increased frequency schedule, the salts readings in your soil should rise.

Also check the pH of your soil slurry with a pH pen. If the pH of your soil is too high, you can flush the soil with pH 7 balanced pure water and you can reduce the pH in your garden over time through subsequent waterings and feedings with a lower level of pH about 5–6. If the pH in your soil is too low (under 5), you can flush it with a deep watering of pure water and you should increase the pH over the next several feedings and waterings to about 8 on your pH pen. When soil readings have returned to normal, begin feeding plants again on a regular schedule and balance water and fertilizer to a perfect 7 on the pH meter. Take a soil slurry reading every month and at the first sign of any growth problems or yellowing of the plants.

Watering

Watering techniques are simple for container systems — when the soil dries out to about a third of the way down the container, water them. Usually, you will water your garden on scheduled days once or twice a week, but don't wait until the plants are too dry. Lift each plant container before watering to determine how much water to give. Since plants use water at different rates, some will need more than others. If the container is light, give it lots of water. Give as much as the plant will take without water running out of the container's drainage holes and overflowing the tray. Water lightly on the first go round — just enough to wet the soil at the top of the container. Then wait 15 minutes for the soil to expand to the sides of the container. Then water again. This deep watering allows the water to be absorbed into the center of the root ball without uselessly running down the inside of the container and into the tray. In a five-gallon plant pot, I normally water with one half gallon of water on the first round and a second half gallon on the second round. This deep watering method can also be used when fertilizing your plants.

I prefer using a hose, a submersible sump pump, and a wand for watering rather than lifting heavy buckets. The sump pump attaches to one end of your hose and drops into the 30- to 50-gallon watering container in your grow room. The wand attaches to the other end of the hose and is used for reaching faraway plants. I remove any spray heads from the wand using a hacksaw because I want only a soft, smooth flow of water that does not take as long as a spray nozzle does to fill the plant pots. I plug the power cord for the sump pump into a switched extension cord so I can turn the water flow on and off by flipping a switch. I always recommend wearing rubber-soled shoes to avoid any shocks on bare feet when using the power cord. With so much water in the room, some inevitably hits the concrete floor, and water can conduct some electricity into your feet when you switch on the power for the sump pump. Remove the sump pump from the water tank when not in use. Leaving it in the water all the time can ruin the seals. Whenever you use the sump pump to deliver food to the plants, rinse it afterward with fresh water to prevent damage to the seals. Just drop the sump pump in the fresh water and run it for a few seconds until the nutrients are flushed away.

If you notice any of your plants wilting between waterings, just top them up with water and don't change the watering schedule of your entire garden. Some plants need more water than others, and some are missed on occasion during the watering cycle due to the effects of good reefer and just plain forgetfulness. Usually, the largest and strongest plants need the most water.

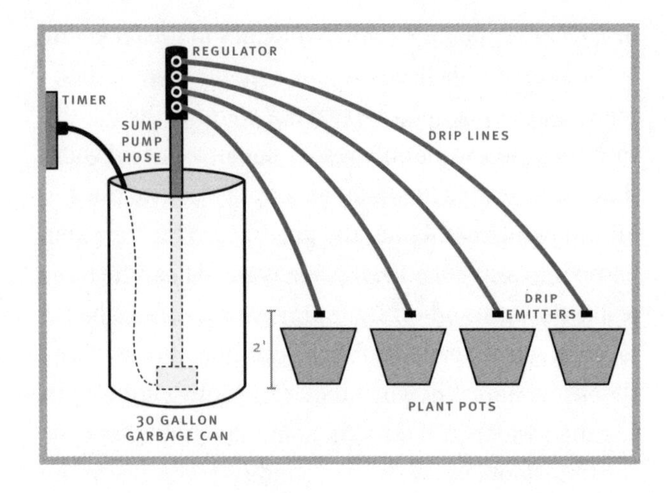

I have also used an outdoor watering timer to water my plants. The electronic timer is run by two aa batteries, which means it is not subject to electrical power interruptions. And this means the timer can be trusted to turn on and off over a given cycle if you want to go away on business trips or vacations. It takes a little practice to get the exact water flow rate by adjusting the tap, but after a few tries it becomes easy. The timer is connected to a hose that runs from the water tap to the grow room. Connect the grow room side of the hose to another piece of plastic hose called a manifold. Drip emitters are plugged into the manifold and feed water through ¼"-thick individual plastic lines that run to each plant pot in the grow room. A visit to any hydroponics shop can provide you with the parts and expertise needed for setting up this type of drip line.

The drip line and timer setup should be used only for pure water, not for delivering hydroponics food to the plants. I recommend hydroponics fertilizers because they are the purest available and will not burn the plants like regular fertilizers, but even hydroponics nutrients will plug up the narrow lines and drip emitters over time. By hand watering and feeding, you can deliver the hydroponics food to just the plants that need it and avoid the ones that don't. With a hydroponics drip system, all of the plants in the garden receive the same nutrients, even those that should not, such as plants almost ready for harvest or very young transplants. Hand feeding is still best.

A day or two after watering or fertilizing your container plants, use your fingers or a small rake to till the top few inches of soil in the pots. This breaks apart the crust that forms when the soil begins to dry out after watering, allowing the free exchange of air and gases that otherwise become trapped within the soil. The crust also causes a slower evaporation of the water from the soil, which results in a longer drying period between waterings which all translates into slower growth in your plants. While you break up the crust that forms on top of the plant pots, also run your finger around the inside top of the pot where the soil becomes compact. Breaking up this soil closes the gap between soil and container, ensuring that water won't simply run down the sides.

Overwatering and Underwatering

If you overwater your plants, they will tell you. They will show sluggish growth, and the leaves will begin to turn yellow and then brown and then die. The soil will be constantly soggy. You might also find gnat flies in the soil and on the plants. If you happen to overwater, simply pour off the excess from the plant pot and then hold back on watering until the soil is dry to the touch at least a few inches below the surface. Then water and fertilize as usual on a regular two- or three-week cycle.

Usually, only one plant in the garden will show the first signs of underwatering. Look for a plant that is wilted and hanging listlessly compared to the other robust plants. A well-watered plant is firm and strong, with its leaves and branches held high and plump with water. An underwatered plant will look as though it is sick and dying, its branches drooping and the soil will be dry to the touch several inches down. Learn to anticipate the need for water before the plants wilt. If a plant wilts and is given water right away, say within a 24-hour period, it will recover with no ill effects. If a plant is allowed to stay wilted any longer than 24 hours, it might become sickly and never return to full health.

Insects

If you discover insect damage in your garden, buy a magnifying glass to identify which insects are damaging your plants. Once you have determined which pests are infesting your garden you may decide to order predator insects that will eat the offending pests. Although they can keep infestations down to some degree, I have never found predator insects to be effective in totally eradicating pests. As a general principle, check your garden once a week to see if there is any insect damage, searching under the leaves for the rotten little pests. Look for tiny spots or white specks on the leaves where the insects have been sucking the juices out of your plants. Look for any movement on the leaves as tiny insects fly or run away from you. Spider mites will spin webs in your plants if they breed heavily. If that ever happens you must remove the webs by hand before attempting any insect controls or treatments.

There are many insecticides on the market, but every time you take a chance with a new insecticide you risk killing or setting back your plants. Some insecticides kill pests. Other insecticides kill both pests and plants. When cannabis plants are in flower, there is almost nothing you can do to eradicate insects that won't hurt your plants. Best to pick the insects off by hand and then let nature take its course. Flowering plants are never far from harvest, and the best treatment for flowering plants with insect infestations is to pull them out of your garden when they are ripe or even a bit earlier and treat only the vegetating plants. Under-ripe marijuana can still be smoked and can provide a worthwhile buzz, although it is neither as sweet nor as potent as a fully developed plant.

I have a foolproof organic insecticide formula that kills all insects without harming my plants. It works on spider mites, thrips, gnats, and white flies, to mention a few of the most common indoor garden pests. Its active ingredient is Einstein oil, which is basically neem oil, from the neem tree, mixed with pyrethrums, which are made from chrysanthemums. Add a few drops of Safer's Insecticidal Soap to the Einstein oil to help the solution stick to the plants. Einstein oil and Safer's Insecticidal Soap are available at most hydroponics stores and garden supply stores and can be ordered online. Do not spray plants at the same time you fertilize, and remember, only spray cannabis in the vegetative cycle.

To make my all-natural insecticide, **you'll need:**

- ☐ 1 teaspoon Einstein oil
- ☐ 2–3 drops of Safer's Insecticidal Soap
- ☐ 4 ¼ cups water
- ☐ spray bottle or pressure sprayer

Then:

1. Add a few drops of Safer's Insecticidal Soap to the water.
2. Shake the room temperature Einstein oil vigorously and then mix with the soap and water solution.
3. Pour solution into spray bottle.
4. Shake the solution repeatedly and do so regularly while using.
5. Spray the soil and wet the undersides of the leaves more than the tops.
6. Wait 10 days and spray again.
7. Keep repeating this cycle until all insects are gone.

This solution won't hurt your plants. It is not so much the quantity or strength of the solution that you deliver to the plants that works – it is the repetition every 10 days. The first spray keeps the insects from breeding and kills most of the adults but does not damage the eggs. The eggs usually hatch within 10 days, so that is why you have to repeat the spraying cycle every 10 days. It might take several weeks or even months before every insect is eradicated, but eventually you'll win the battle even if your plants were overrun with insects.

Yellow sticky cards are an excellent means of trapping insects and alerting you to pests. They can be purchased at any garden store, and as a general rule, I place a number of the sticky cards in with my vegetating plants but not so many in with my flowering plants.

If you use an air conditioner, insects are less likely to cause problems in your garden. They prefer warm, humid climates to breed in. Air-conditioned grow rooms are cool and dry like laboratories – a hostile environment for bugs and an excellent climate for keeping indoor plants healthy. Insects are attracted to weakened plants under stress, and air conditioners prevent plant stress.

When you discover insects, determine how they entered your garden in the first place, and plug that leak into your grow room. Then treat the insects as described above. To learn more about recognizing insects and insect damage, go to the library or research online for more photos and details.

Diseases

Diseases are occasional visitors to the indoor garden, and there are many known and unknown pathogens that can kill your plants or stunt their growth. Root rot. Fungal infections. Leaf spot. Disease is often brought into a sterile room on the soles of outdoor shoes and on dirty garden tools and other equipment. It stands to reason, then, that you shouldn't share your cannabis garden tools with any other plants outside your grow room. If used equipment is brought into the grow room, it should be sterilized in bleach solution first. Also be sure to always use sterilized soil, so diseases aren't carried from the outdoors to the plants.

Even if all the proper protocols are followed, insects can still carry diseases into your indoor garden, thereby infecting the plants. To treat any disease you find, clean and sterilize your room and then remove any infected plants and replace them with fresh, healthy plants. Don't bother with fungicides for root rot or leaf spot or plant virus. Even when fungicides work the plants are often left permanently weakened by disease or virus. In extreme cases you might have to kill all your plants (including clones) and start a new garden from fresh seeds, although it is rare to have to go to such lengths. Usually, disease is aggravated by humid growing conditions, which cause your glasses to fog up when you enter the grow room. If that happens, install more vent fans or an air conditioner and everything will improve. For information on specific plant ailments, go to the library or on the Internet.

A good general principle when treating plants for any problem — whether it is overwatering, underwatering, insects, diseases, over- or underfertilization, high or low pH — is to be patient. Plants take a long time to react, so do not expect changes overnight and don't keep pumping in the antidote to the problem. Go slow. Take time. Whenever there is a choice between doing too much or doing too little — choose doing too little.

Garden Maintenance Checklist

I suggest visiting your budding room and your vegetative room for a few minutes every day, just to keep an eye on problems before they become unmanageable. Use your five senses to discover problems. You will smell any electrical burning, plant ripeness, or plant rot in your room. You will hear any squeaks, squeals, and other strange noises from your grow equipment. Your eyes will alert you to plant health, insects, and lamp strength or burnouts. You will feel any heat buildup in the room. And your sense of taste will alert you to how well you have grown your product in the final test.

Aside from the feeding and watering we've already discussed, there are several tasks that should be done on a daily, weekly, or monthly basis. Use a calendar to keep track of feeding schedules and other information, such as breeding characteristics or individual plant health. Use plant tags that you stick into the soil to assign plant names or numbers to the plants in order to keep track of different species. The following checklist will help you keep track of tasks until you check them automatically.

Checklist

DAILY

- ☐ Pick off any dead growth on plants
- ☐ Look for insect damage on plants, or insects around lights or in the room
- ☐ Look for signs of fertilizer damage on plants
- ☐ Check room temperature and humidity
- ☐ Check soil moisture

WEEKLY

- ☐ Check pH in water reservoir and adjust if necessary
- ☐ Stake plants with bamboo and bend tips if they are growing tall
- ☐ Rotate plants around the room so they get the desired amount of light

MONTHLY

- ☐ Check vent timers and light timers to ensure they're working properly
- ☐ Re-check timers if any adjustments are made
- ☐ Test pH and salts pens to ensure accuracy
- ☐ Test salts and pH levels in soil with a slurry solution
- ☐ Check air conditioning filters for dust build-up and clean as required
- ☐ Empty air conditioning water reservoir if necessary
- ☐ Turn off lamps, let them cool, and clean lamps and vented hood glass with vinegar and water or glass cleaner
- ☐ Vacuum and wash floors of grow room

BIANNUALLY

- ☐ Change all lightbulbs

ANNUALLY

- ☐ Change charcoal filters
- ☐ Buy new pH and salts testing solutions
- ☐ Change batteries in pH pen and salts pen
- ☐ Buy new hormone rooting powder

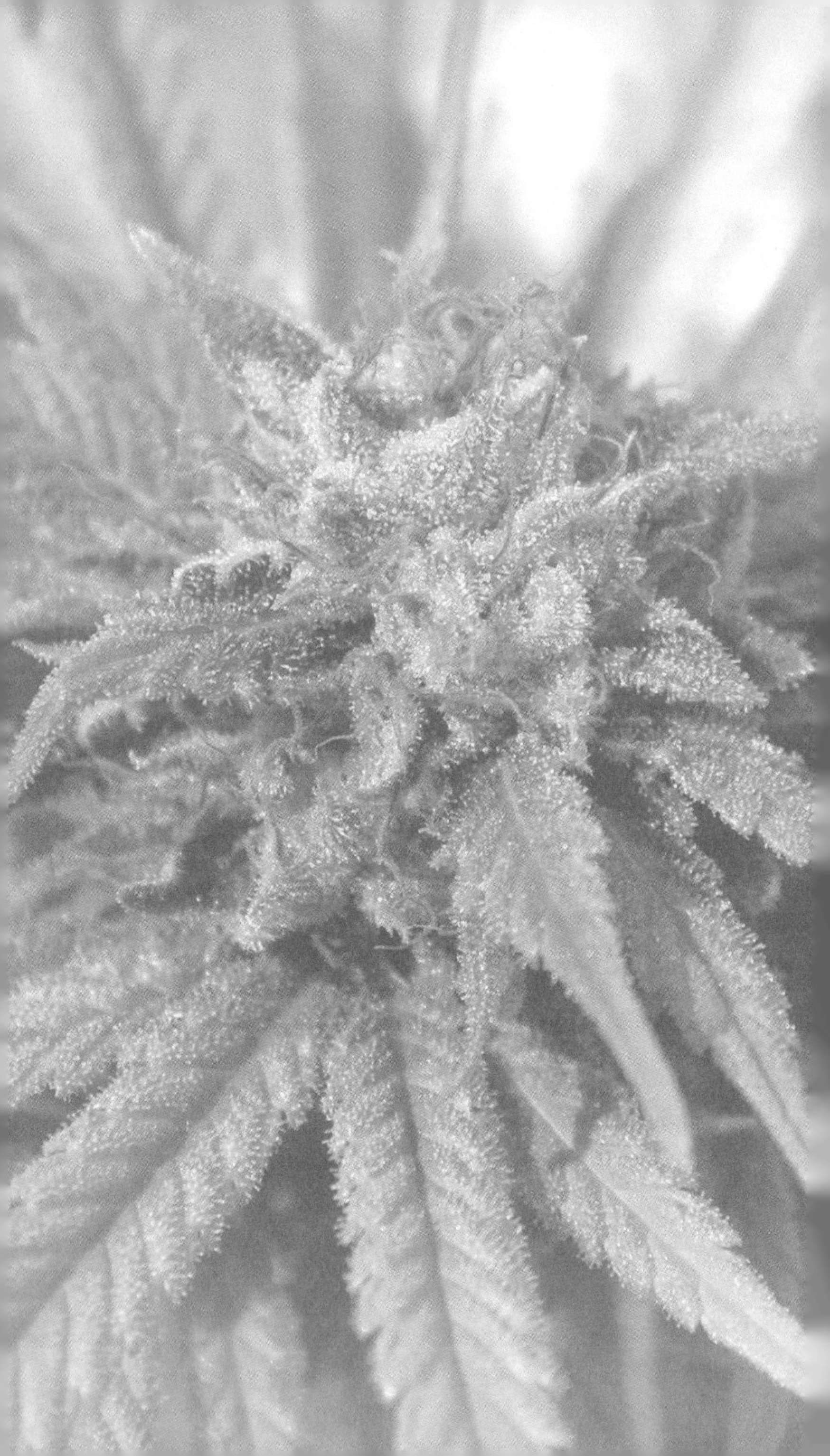

4

REAPING *Your* HARVEST

Turnaround Time

Harvest time is also called turnaround time, since it's when one crop comes to an end and a new crop begins. As I've explained, every two months you'll need to rotate your plants: harvesting plants finished their budding phase, transplanting vegetative plants to the budding room, and cloning new plants. Here are the basic steps for that important transition:

1. Cut plants for harvest and hang to dry or begin curing process (read on for details).
2. Empty soil medium and drainage rocks from five-gallon pots into trash bag for disposal.
3. Flush the lava rock residue remaining in the plant pots in the yard or garage (to avoid clogging drains).
4. Sterilize containers with a water and bleach solution of about one cup of bleach per two gallons of water.
5. Add about 2" of fresh drainage rocks to sterilized five-gallon containers, then fill containers halfway with fresh soilless mix.
6. Transplant vegetative plants to large containers, and then fill pots with soilless mix to about 2" below the rim. Follow these steps again for one-gallon vegetative containers to prepare them for new clones.

Sterilization between crops is crucial. You can break that rule a few times and get away with it, but if you don't sterilize your plant containers and tools between every crop you risk getting a virus or disease or pest that can destroy your entire harvest — all because you were too lazy or undisciplined to follow the correct protocols.

Harvesting Cannabis

Once the cannabis plant is ready for harvest, it must be cut down and dried. The time to harvest plants is when the buds become full and sticky with resin. If the top buds feel hard when you squeeze them, instead of soft and pliable, they are ready for harvest. (Don't squeeze them *too* often because it damages the white hairs and THC glands and retards bud development.) Do not try squeezing lower buds because they often seem soft even when the plant is mature. Another sign of a mature cannabis plant is when the white hairs that split out of the flower pods turn red or brown. For the best view of the resin glands/crystals, use a 15-power magnifying glass. Resin glands start as pointed capitates, like a stiletto, and when the glands are mature they will develop fat heads. The heads are a clear transparent color when juvenile and turn cloudy or opaque when fully mature or overripe. Harvest when the majority of resin glands are still clear to obtain perfectly developed buds. Practice all of these methods for timing your harvest, and of course use your nose to smell the delightful scent of a mature cannabis flower/bud. If the plant is mature in all of the above tests and there is no scent, you have probably waited too long to harvest.

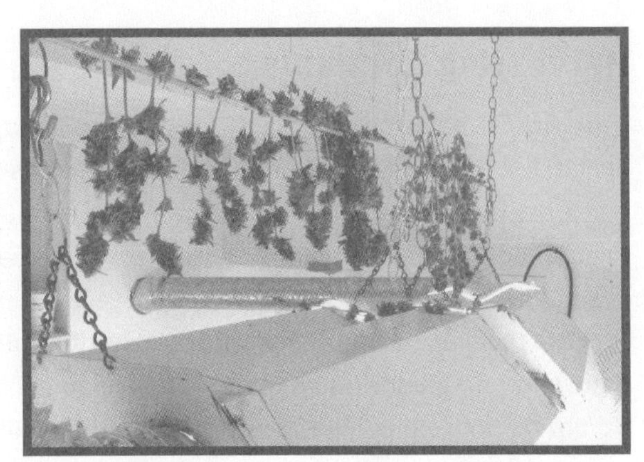

Cannabis buds hanging to dry above grow lights

If you remember from the beginning of this book, it is resin glands or crystals that you are growing, not the plant material itself. Any part of the plant with a heavy coating of crystals is the part you want to keep. Usually just the buds are taken but there is some smokable crystal that can be harvested from associated leaf that surrounds the buds. Any green parts that don't have crystals should be trimmed off and discarded. Those parts of the plant offer no THC, and they make the buds taste bitter when smoked.

Cutting your plants is the stinkiest time of all, so if you are concerned about odors you must compensate for them. You can use aerosol deodorizers or put some fabric softener sheets in the dryer. Brew some coffee. Bake some bread. Fry up some bacon. Do anything you can to mitigate the smell of freshly cut skunk weed. If you have properly sealed and vented your grow room, it is an excellent place to cut up your weed. The smells will stay in the room and be vented through a carbon filter or ozone generator to your catch basin, be it a chimney, garage, attic, window, or whatever. Whether you are cutting a large amount or a small amount of herb, pick your time well so that no one comes to your front door. If someone does, don't answer it.

Here are the basic steps to drying your weed:

1. Remove all of the buds from the plant.
2. Trim each branch and remove excess green leaf from the buds.
3. Crisscross wires over your hooded lamp reflectors and hang the buds on the wires, or hang a screen horizontally over the lamp hoods and lay the buds on the screen.
4. Leave the weed to dry for a minimum of three to four days. In about seven days, the buds will begin to taste better. In 10 days, they can be stored in a baggie, although a glass jar is better for long-term storage.

Purists say you should dry your plants with the leaves on and trim the plants only after they are dry. But that is messy and in my opinion not worth the effort; I have never been able to taste any difference in drying plants this way if the buds were of good quality to start with.

Curing Your Buds

While you can smoke your bud with a basic drying method, to get the best out of your plant, you should also cure it. Cured buds taste smoother and milder than dried buds, and they are preferred by cannabis aficionados.

To cure your weed:

1. Follow the regular steps for drying your bud.
2. Place buds in a baggie or sealed glass jar and leave them to sweat for one or two days.
3. When you remove the buds, they will be damp again. Place them to dry over your grow room lights again for 24 hours.
4. Return buds to the plastic or glass container.
5. Check the buds after one or two days to see if they seem damp; repeat the process of sweating and drying until they no longer feel or smell damp. When the bud branches snap rather than bend, the buds can be put away for any length of time in any kind of container, and they won't incur any rot or bad taste.

After a month or more in storage, the buds can be considered cured and will taste the best they can for months and even years to come. Cured cannabis loses its green color and becomes the more familiar brown shades reminiscent of outdoor weed.

Rub It Out

My Jamaican friends showed me a trick for improving the taste and burning qualities of freshly harvested weed. When cannabis is very fresh to the point of dampness it is usually cut up with scissors in order to roll a joint without the pot clumping into a mound of wet leaf that does not burn well. Instead of using scissors, try placing the damp weed into the palm of your hand and use the palm of your other hand to grind and mash the cannabis bud into little bits. It takes a few minutes, but the results are well worth the effort. By mashing the weed with one hand into the palm of the other, you effectively grind the resin on the surface of the fresh leaf deep into the leaf itself. Even the sweetest cannabis leaf is a little bitter and burns poorly until it dries out, but this process will sweeten up the bitter taste of the leaf and improve the burnability of the not yet dry weed by blending it with oily THC resin glands. In a side by side comparison test, you will find a dramatic improvement in the flavor and burnability of fresh cannabis joints after "rubbing out" your uncured smoke.

Breeding

Breeding plants is a hobby for the advanced cannabis grower who wants her pot to be all it should be. My best weed has always been the weed I bred myself. Often that dynamite cannabis came from two lesser strains. To breed cannabis, you must place a male plant beside a female plant so the pollen from the male flowers pollinates the female flowers and makes new seeds that possess traits of both parents. The seeds from a pollinated plant will vary widely, with some producing dynamite plants and some producing lesser plants. It is a simple matter to throw out the crappy plants that are stunted or smoke harshly and keep the good ones for your garden by cloning. Only one plant is required to give you hundreds of seeds. Do not try to pollinate a plant in your grow room unless you want the entire crop to be pollinated. Even if you sprinkle a tiny bit of pollen over one single plant in your grow room, the pollen will scatter and fertilize most of the other plants in the room.

Usually, the female plant is available from your personal garden. You must buy seeds to get a male plant because, unless a grower is breeding, male plants are usually thrown out as soon as they are identified. Once you have a male plant and a female plant, **follow these simple steps to create new custom marijuana strains:**

1. As soon as the male flowers, it should be taken out of the budding room and kept alive by natural lights or grow lights. A flowering female plant should also be removed from the budding room. The male and female plants must be covered if necessary to keep them in a 12-hour light/dark regimen.
2. Place a dark page of a glossy magazine under the male plant. When you see that yellow pollen has dropped from the plant onto the magazine page, it is time to place the two plants together.
3. Put the plants as close to each other as possible and gently shake the male plant to release its pollen over the female plant.
4. Pollinate the female several times a day for a couple of days, and then dispose of the male plant in your private yard or compost pile. (Not your garbage can — unless you are looking to get busted.)
5. Sprinkle any pollen on the magazine page over the female plant.
6. Place the female back in the budding room. Hopefully, you can do so before any pests from outside settle onto the plant and get carried into the grow room.

The female plant will begin showing swollen seed pods within a few weeks. A few weeks after the seed pods swell, the seeds will begin breaking open from their husks and will turn from white to yellow and finally to dark brown. When the plant is ready to harvest, the seeds will be dark and waxy and ready to germinate.

The best way to de-seed dried marijuana is to break up the buds and use a magazine or any other rough surface to roll the seeds away from the bud bits. Newspaper is not recommended for this task if you intend to smoke any of the weed bits that are left behind on the magazine. The newspaper ink will make the smoke taste bitter and is not very good for human consumption in any form. Use one hand to lightly sweep the visible seeds into a bowl or onto a table, and use your other hand to shake and vibrate the magazine to free more seeds from the buds. Rotate the magazine as you work so that the seeds are always rolling away from the pot bits. Seeds can be kept many years and even decades if they are dried and stored properly. They should be stored in an airtight container in a cool, dry place.

Vacations

If you are going away for a few days or weeks and want to keep your garden alive, have a trusted friend take care of your room. If you prefer to keep things to yourself, simply bury some water crystals in the soil of your plants before you leave. Water crystals can be purchased at any hydroponics store. They are placed in a bucket of water and become a gel as they absorb many times their weight in moisture. They are then mixed into the soil and provide at least a week of water for growing plants. When using crystals to keep plants alive, turn off extra grow room lights so that the temperature is kept as low as possible, thereby causing the plants to use less water.

Another trick is to purchase a garden hose timer, which is available at hardware stores and hydroponics stores. A garden hose with timer attachment is connected to a water faucet that is turned to the open position and the timer will turn the hose on every day or two, for a set period of time, to automatically water the plants. A manifold is plugged into the hose when it reaches the grow room and smaller "spaghetti hoses" run from the manifold to deliver water to the individual plants. It takes some practice beforehand to learn the correct settings, but once set up timers can water a garden over a period of weeks. I don't suggest this method of watering anywhere other than a concrete basement with a floor drain in case the timer fails. A safer method of automatic watering uses a reservoir that holds a limited amount of water, say 30 or 40 gallons, such as a plastic garbage can. A regular hydroponics watering pump on a timer can then be used to water plants from the reservoir over a period of days or even weeks. The water pickup in the reservoir should be lower than the drip emitters to prevent any water siphoning down to the plants when the pump turns off.

Light timers should be set as usual and will turn off and on repeatedly while you are gone. Timers must be the type that will turn on again automatically after a power failure. To minimize the need for watering the plants, don't use an air conditioner or dehumidifier during your absence and set your grow room to cool itself with vent fans only. Turn off unnecessary grow lights while you are away to keep the room as cool as possible, which will keep the plants dormant to some degree. The plants will resume vigorous growth when you return from vacation and turn up the lighting to full strength.

If none of these methods is appealing, you can always shut down your garden and restart it with clones kept alive in your living room along with your other house plants. House plants live in a continual dormant state and need far less water than cannabis plants in a grow room. If you are uncomfortable with leaving cannabis clones around your house or apartment, you can always restart your garden with seeds. Seeds are preferred to clones that have been taken from diseased or damaged plants.

Troubleshooting

Lights don't turn on?

Check the timer first to make sure it is set correctly and operating as it should. Then try plugging your lamp directly into a socket without using the timer. If the light turns on, then only the timer needs replacing. If the light doesn't turn on, check the circuit breaker in the main panel. If the problem isn't in the main panel, check if you need a new lightbulb. If a new lightbulb doesn't do the trick, take the ballast and lamp reflector into a hydroponics store for examination and repair and replace if necessary.

Fan stopped working?

Verify that the timer is working properly. Make sure the fan and timer are plugged in properly. Check the circuit breaker in the main panel. Replace the fan or timer with a new one.

Odor building up in the house?

Check that vent fans are operating correctly and vent hoses are connected properly. Ensure that the air conditioner is working. Is it plugged in? Is the water reservoir full? Does the intake or exhaust filter need to be cleaned? Is the glass closed tightly on the vented lamp hoods? If the vented air circulation is becoming weak or slow, you might have to buy a new carbon air filter. As a preventative measure, replace the filter every year.

Heat building up in the room?

Verify that vent fans are operating and vent hoses are connected properly. Check the air conditioner. Is it plugged in and turned on? Is the water reservoir full? Does the intake or exhaust filter need to be cleaned? Is the glass closed tightly on the vented lamp hoods? If a vent fan is blowing weakly, you might have to buy a new carbon air filter.

Plants growing slowly?

Check the age of your grow lamps and change the bulbs every six months without fail. Are the grow lights the correct distance from the plants? Is the room the correct temperature and humidity? Remember, the ideal growing temperature is 78–80 degrees Fahrenheit, and the ideal blooming humidity is 50–60 percent. The ideal vegetative humidity is 60–70 percent. Don't be alarmed if your temperature is a few degrees higher than 80. High humidity is more of a concern than high temperature. A grow room should never be higher than 80 percent humidity. Perform a soil slurry to assess your soil's pH and salts levels. Check for pests.

Plants looking sick?

Look for pests. Check for too much or too little water in soil. Examine leaves for signs of overfertilizing and roots for yellowing or disease. Smell the roots for the pleasant odor of fresh potatoes rather than the unpleasant odor of sour soil. Check your room temperature and humidity over a 24-hour period. When in doubt about the health of your garden, always perform a soil slurry to check pH and salts/fertilizer levels.

Salts pen or pH pen not working or giving erratic readings?

Test the pen batteries and change them if required. Use fine sandpaper to clean the electronic prongs and absorbent cloth to clean the glass bubble at the bottom of the pens. Buy a fresh test solution and retest pens.